VAN BU~~~~~ W9-BKT-617
DECATUR. MICHIGAN 49045

Second Edition of *Kids with Celiac Disease*

GLUTEN-FREE KIDS

Raising Happy, Healthy Children with Ceiliac Disease, Autism, and Other Conditions

Danna Korn

DISCARDED

Woodbine House ◆ 2010

618.9239
Kor

© 2001, 2010 Danna Korn
Revised edition

All rights reserved. Published in the United States of American by Woodbine House, 6510 Bells Mill Road, Bethesda, MD 20817. 800-843-7323. www.woodbinehouse.com.

This book is a revised and expanded edition of *Kids with Celiac Disease: A Family Guide to Raising Happy, Healthy, Gluten-Free Children* by Danna Korn (Woodbine House, 2001).

Library of Congress Cataloging-in-Publication Data

Korn, Danna.
  Gluten-free kids : raising happy, healthy children with celiac disease, autism, and other conditions / by Danna Korn. -- Rev. ed.
       p. cm.
  Rev. ed. of: Kids with celiac disease / Danna Korn.
  Includes index.
  ISBN 978-1-60613-006-3(trade pbk.)
 1. Celiac disease--Diet therapy. 2. Gluten-free diet. 3. Children--Diseases--Treatment.
I. Korn, Danna. Kids with celiac disease. II. Title.
  RJ456.C44K67 2010
  618.92'399--dc22

2010030028

Manufactured in the United States of America

10 9 8 7 6 5 4 3 2 1

10/11
BdT

Dedication

This book is dedicated to those who inspire positive attitudes, even in the face of adversity.

"You can complain because roses have thorns, or you can rejoice because thorns have roses."

—Ziggy

"When I hear somebody sigh, 'Life is hard,' I am always tempted to ask, 'Compared to what?'"

—Sydney Harris

"Life consists not in holding good cards but in playing those you hold well."
—Josh Billings

"Destiny is not a matter of chance, it is a matter of choice; it is not a thing to be waited for, it is a thing to be achieved."

—William Jennings Bryan

"The problem is not that there are problems. The problem is expecting otherwise and thinking that having problems is a problem."

—Theodore Rubin

While there is really no need to explain the relevance of these analogies to those of us who are raising gluten-free kids, I hope everyone who reads this book will make the connection and guide their children toward an optimistic, productive, happy, healthy, gluten-free future.

Table of Contents

About the Author

Known as "The Gluten-Free Guru," Danna Korn is an author, motivational speaker, and renowned expert in the wellness industry. She is the author of six books, all on the subject of living and loving a gluten-free lifestyle. Respected as one of the leading authorities on the gluten-free diet and the medical conditions that benefit from it, she has been featured in *People* magazine, on ABC's *20-20*, and dozens of other national media outlets.

Danna began her career as a gluten-free pioneer in 1991, when her son, Tyler, was diagnosed with celiac disease, a genetic intolerance to gluten. Doctors told her that her son, like others with celiac disease, would "suffer" a life of deprivation and restrictions, and they gave her no direction for following a gluten-free diet, which was the key to his improved health. Danna wasn't about to accept that Tyler would have to "suffer" or "cope," nor would she flounder like many others attempting a gluten-free diet did. Furthermore, she was committed to helping others who could benefit from her knowledge. She was a mom on a mission to help millions. (You can read more about Danna's story of Tyler's diagnosis in the introduction to this book.)

Without the benefit of the Internet (it hadn't been invented yet), and ignoring the widespread warnings that no one would ever publish a book on the subject, Danna conducted extensive medical research with the nation's foremost experts, and then wrote her first book—she sent four proposals to publishers. She received four acceptances, including one from Woodbine House to publish what would be her first book, *Kids with Celiac Disease*. Her work in the gluten-free community has had profound effects, resulting in availability of products that would never have made it to store shelves without her influence with retailers and manufacturers.

Six books and thousands of speaking engagements later, Danna has earned the reputation of being a guru in the world of gluten "freedom"—and in the process has helped improve the lives of millions by helping them adopt a healthier lifestyle.

She founded and runs the world's largest support group of its type, R.O.C.K. (Raising Our Celiac Kids), which has more than 140 chapters throughout the U.S. and Canada. She also consults or has consulted for companies including General Mills, Whole Foods, Hain-Celestial, and Prometheus Laboratories.

Danna's passion for wellness extends far beyond gluten-free living. She is co-founder, Chief Executive Officer, and Chief Motivational Officer of Sonic Boom Wellness, an innovative corporate wellness company with more than 100 well-known clients throughout the U.S. and Canada.

Acknowledgements

When I decided to write my first book about raising gluten-free kids, it was solely for the purpose of helping others. In a lonely world with no Internet, no kids' support groups, no others dealing with what I was dealing with, it felt right to reach out and help people if I could.

So I wrote a few chapters of *Kids with Celiac Disease,* but was warned by just about everyone I talked to, "No one will publish your book. No one has even *heard* of celiac disease." And I had never gotten a book published—something most people hinted was nearly an impossibility.

But the people at Woodbine House were willing to talk to me, and eventually agreed to publish what would become my first of six books on the subject of living (and loving) the gluten-free lifestyle.

Several years, hundreds of speaking engagements, dozens of magazine articles and TV appearances, and a bunch of books later, I am fortunate to have met thousands of people who have told me I've made a difference in their lives. That is what life is all about.

To the people at Woodbine House who gave me my first shot at living a dream of helping others, thank you. To the many leaders in the gluten-free community from whom I've learned so much, thank you. To the people who have taken the time to let me know that my work in the gluten-free community has helped improve their lives—thank you—because that's what this is all about.

And it seems so obvious that it doesn't need to be said, but it should be: thank you to my son, Tyler; my daughter, Kelsie; and my husband, Bryan, for your undying love and ubiquitous support for everything I do, even when it seems (or is) a little crazy.

Foreword
By Jenny McCarthy

When you're planning a family, you don't think about celiac disease, food sensitivities, autism, or any other life-altering condition. You dream of a healthy, happy child who will have every advantage in life. But when your child is diagnosed with a condition that changes the lives of every member of the family, those dreams are shattered, or at least they take a different form.

When my son was first diagnosed with autism, I was like most parents of autistic kids—stunned. One of the most frustrating aspects is that so little is known about autism, and even medical professionals will often admit that treatment options are, at best, limited. Most parents are told that there's little or nothing that can be done—they're advised to accept the situation and move on.

The truth is, there are a lot of treatment protocols showing promise for autism, including the gluten-free/casein-free diet. I realize there are skeptics out there who do not acknowledge that the diet may be a viable treatment option—but many of us have tried it and have seen remarkable improvements in our children. We embrace the improvements we see and we take pride in forging a better life for our children.

It isn't easy. We work hard to educate our kids' caretakers and friends and family. We endure the tantrums, and comfort our kids when they want to eat what all the other kids are eating. Simple social situations can turn into culinary nightmares. Following the diet is a lot of work, but it's well worth it. If you're raising a gluten-free child or considering putting your child on a gluten-free diet, *Gluten-Free Kids* is a must-read. This is Danna's sixth book on living—and loving—the gluten-free lifestyle. Danna dove into the deep end of the gluten-free pool in 1991 when her son was diagnosed with celiac disease. Since then she has earned kudos from some of the world's foremost researchers on the gluten-free diet and medical conditions that benefit from it, and is today known as The Gluten-Free Guru. While her books are helpful for people adopting the gluten-free lifestyle at any age, her passion is helping parents raise happy, healthy, gluten-free kids, and that passion leaps off every page of her books.

Danna's books take you beyond just the diet. As parents of gluten-free kids, we have emotional and social issues that go beyond the food itself—and the kids have issues to deal with, too. Danna gets it. She's "been there-done that," raising a gluten-free son and adopting the gluten-free lifestyle herself. The founder of R.O.C.K. (Raising Our Celiac Kids), she provides tremendous insight into the issues families face in a gluten-free lifestyle through experience, research, humor, and optimism.

Whether you're looking for help with the diet, medical and scientific information, or a sanguine perspective on how to deal with the emotional and social implications of raising a gluten-free child, *Gluten-Free Kids* is indispensable.

Introduction:
This Book—What It Is
and What It Isn't

"I want readers to know that I'm not just an author. I'm a mom who, on a mission to save my son, had to learn the hard way how to raise a happy, healthy, gluten-free kid. If I can share what I've learned and spare others the fear and confusion I felt at one time, I will feel forever privileged."

—Danna Korn

There are lots of reasons people are considering or embarking upon a gluten-free lifestyle for their children. Many of you aren't only eliminating gluten, but cutting out casein, too. Adapting to a new lifestyle like this means an entirely new way of life that encompasses much more than "simply" a dietary change. It's huge. It means you'll have to think before driving through a fast food restaurant; you'll need to make special accommodations for birthday parties and outings; you'll need to educate just about everyone who ever comes in contact with your child. And, at least at first, it will seem as though there is *nothing* your child can eat. If the idea of all of this is still fresh for you, and, perhaps, even if it isn't, you're most likely experiencing myriad emotions, ranging from panic to hysteria, confusion, and relief.

I know you want to skip to the end where I tell you the magic key to making it all easier, but reading these preliminaries should be worthwhile. If nothing else, you will find out that I can empathize. My son has celiac disease—believe me, I know what you're going through.

To those of you embarking upon the gluten-free lifestyle because your child has been diagnosed with autism or other conditions on the autism spectrum, I applaud you. There are lots of skeptics out there, but it's a brave, bold move you're making with potentially profound effects. Please forgive me if it seems that much of this book is devoted to parents of kids with gluten sensitivity or celiac disease. That's where my experience lies. Yet I believe in the opportunity you have to improve your kids' lives. I have therefore expanded the scope of this book from its original focus on kids with celiac disease so that it also offers advice that will help you raise happy, healthy, and gluten-free/casein-free kids.

Regardless of your reason for reading this book, I sincerely hope that it will simplify your life, help you deal with day-to-day situations, show you how to provide the most supportive emotional environment for your child, give you an optimistic outlook on your child's future, and comfort you when you feel that no one understands. Oh—and by the way—it really *does* get easier!

Why I Wrote This Book

My son was diagnosed with celiac disease when he was 18 months old. Prior to the diagnosis, we had the same story many of you have had: a child with 20 diarrhea diapers a day; huge, distended belly, skinny arms, lack of energy; and visits to several insensitive doctors who had no idea what was *really* wrong, but had the gall to tell me, with that condescending, why-are-you-wasting-my-time-I-have-real-patients-waiting tone,

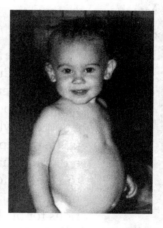

Nothing wrong?! Tyler had a distended belly and more than a dozen diarrhea diapers a day, and was lethargic and irritable. Yet three pediatricians told us there was nothing to be concerned about and sent us away.

that there was nothing wrong with my child. One pediatrician actually took my hand, and with a kind, but patronizing smile, said, "I know, honey. Mommies get really neurotic about diarrhea. It won't last forever, you know." But of course—why hadn't I realized that it was *my* neurosis that was resulting in the 20 diarrhea diapers a day?

Nine months and three doctors later, I was still apparently neurotic. When our insurance changed and we were forced to go to a new pediatric group, I thought nothing of dragging in a listless, lethargic baby with skinny arms and legs and a belly that begged for not-so-amusing jokes about a pregnant toddler. By then, tired of being told there was nothing wrong with my child, I had resigned myself to the fact that I must have just gotten one of those kids who poops a lot, and I sure wasn't going to talk about it any further, for fear *everyone* would then know how neurotic I had actually been. So when, during a routine ear check, the new pediatrician expressed concern about Tyler's distended belly, I broke down and cried, thankful that finally someone was going to believe that there really *was* something wrong with my son.

You can probably guess what we went through next. Daily visits to the hospital, working with the pediatric gastroenterologist to rule out everything from cystic fibrosis to cancer to a rare blood disorder. A week later, when he suggested that we do a biopsy and check for yet another disease we had never heard of—celiac disease—we numbly nodded our approval and signed yet another release form. Several months and three biopsies later, we had our confirmation. The good news was that there was a label for what was wrong with our son. The bad news was that it was going to require more than a few changes in our lives. A bittersweet diagnosis, indeed.

My Son's Diagnosis—What Now?

Keep in mind, this all took place long before Al Gore had invented the Internet. There were no support groups for gluten-free kids; there weren't always toll-free numbers on packaging; food labeling laws hadn't been passed, so labels were confusing and uninformative. I was terrified to feed my own child!

For the first three days after Tyler was diagnosed with celiac disease, he ate nothing but French fries and Fritos. I was scared to death I was going to poison him. I got brave and decided to head to my local grocery store—after all, I'm an intelligent person—how hard could it be to read a few labels? Two hours later, I left with tear-stained cheeks and four bags of Fritos.

Thinking quickly and pulling myself together, I headed to the local health food store. Thankfully, they actually carried frozen loaves of gluten-free bread! I choked at the nearly $5 per-loaf price tag (today it's more like $7), but remembering it was for my baby boy, I cheerfully bought five loaves and headed home with a renewed sense of optimism.

I covered a piece of toast with jelly and nearly cried with joy as I handed it to him. Well, I almost handed it to him. Because, as any of you who have bought that stuff know, when you look at it too hard, it falls apart. So I gathered the pieces, "glued" them together with more jelly, and held my breath while I watched him take his first bite of gluten-free bread. He spit that piece of bread so far I was finding pieces of it three days later! Obviously, I was going to have to work on finding some better foods, or even—gasp—make my own!

I realized that what I needed was a little support. So I asked our pediatric gastroenterologist where I could find the local support group for parents of kids with celiac disease. Keep in mind, this was in 1991, so you may be able to predict the next part: "The what?" There was no such group. There *was*, however, a group for adults with celiac disease, and we figured that was just as good.

Still somewhat in shock from the diagnosis, off we went to our first celiac support group. We expected to be greeted with pamphlets and flyers on how to deal with babysitters and other caretakers, going to school, and Halloween and other special occasions.

Please don't misunderstand me here. Those groups are *great*, and I so very much appreciate their hard work (and they've come a *long* way since then). But, while the group we met seemed friendly and knowledgeable, we quickly tired of hearing about which fat-free foods were gluten-free, which senior supplements were gluten-free (the average age of the group was nearly double my own), which Thai restaurants were safe (oh sure, my two-year-old was begging for Thai), and how to prevent weight gain once on a gluten-free diet. It became clear that adults with celiac disease had different concerns than I had. I wanted information I could actually *use,* and I was growing impatient with the lack of pertinent, helpful advice on raising *kids* on a gluten-free diet.

I figured maybe it was the *previous* meeting when all of the parental advice had been given, and I had just missed out. Maybe if I asked the right questions....

So, at the end of the meeting, I eagerly stood up and explained that my baby boy had just been diagnosed, and wondered where I could find the pamphlets on raising kids with celiac disease. Not a word. After an awkward silence, the room began to buzz again with talk of more adult issues, and I realized we were completely alone in our plight. (Thankfully, a lot has changed in the last several years, and these local support groups are now actually quite knowledgeable about raising gluten-free kids!)

R.O.C.K. (Raising Our Celiac Kids) Was Born

It was then, in 1991, that I decided that once we got a handle on things, I'd be there to help other people. So I decided to start a support group for families of kids with celiac disease. I came up with the name R.O.C.K., which stands for Raising Our Celiac Kids, and set out to find people who might want to be included in our group. We contacted our pediatric gastroenterologist, figuring he probably had dozens of families looking for support in raising their celiac kids. He put us in touch with *the* other family that he knew of in San Diego County. With some local publicity and networking with other pediatricians, slowly our membership grew to include several families.

Today, R.O.C.K. is an international support group with hundreds of chapters around the world (see www.celiackids.com or www.gfcfkids.com to find one near you). While R.O.C.K. started as a group for kids with celiac disease, it has expanded to include kids on the gluten-free/casein-free diet, regardless of why they're on the diet. I suppose someday we'll need to change the name, but for now families find their way in and we welcome them. The newbies are easy to spot, as we can hear the fear, the frustration, the panic, and the desperation. And we recognize it because we were there. But soon these parents' worries turn to relief, and they know that they can move on.

Beyond Celiac Disease

In the many years since I originally wrote my first book, *Kids with Celiac Disease,* the number of people putting their kids on a gluten-free diet has skyrocketed, and the reasons are vast. People have learned that a gluten-free (and casein-free) diet may dramatically improve symptoms of autism and attention-deficit disorders. They have realized that there are sensitivities to gluten that are not celiac disease, so even if tests are negative for celiac disease, a gluten-free lifestyle may dramatically improve their child's health. Others are putting children on a gluten-free diet to help with autoimmune conditions, or simply because they feel it's healthier.

Why people are embarking upon these new lifestyles for their kids isn't important to me. What does matter is that this book will help them understand how to raise *happy, healthy* gluten-free (and casein-free) kids.

What This Book Isn't...

It isn't a product guide. In fact, there will be little mention of specific brand names. If we do refer to a commercially sold product or food item, you should always check its status to confirm that it is, in fact, gluten-free, because products and ingredients change; it would be impossible to keep up with every product out there.

This book isn't a cookbook. It isn't a medical guide, and it most definitely is not a panacea for all of the difficult situations you may encounter in raising your child.

What This Book Is...

This book is your guide for raising happy, healthy, gluten-free/casein-free kids. I remember how desperate I was for menu and snack suggestions, so I've included plenty of ideas that will keep your child well-fed. You'll find lists of safe and forbidden ingredients, advice for dealing with social and emotional issues, and everything else you'll need to know. Just when you ask yourself a question about your child's gluten-free lifestyle, you'll find it in this book.

You may want to give this book to your family, teachers, friends, and people with whom your child spends a lot of time. It's important that everyone understand the intricacies of the diet, and in some cases, the need for strict adherence.

But more than anything, this book is intended to help you deal with the unique situations we face as parents of kids on a gluten-free diet:

- ◆ What exactly is gluten?
- ◆ What is casein?
- ◆ How do I know if my child should be gluten-free?
- ◆ Should he be casein-free too?
- ◆ What kinds of tests do we need?
- ◆ What can I do if my doctor doesn't understand?
- ◆ How do I prepare my child for the testing?
- ◆ What does his diagnosis mean?

◆ How do I talk to my family about it?

◆ How do I find out what foods are okay for him?

◆ How do we send him to school without worrying he'll get gluten?

◆ What can I feed him for quick snacks?

◆ What do we do for Halloween and other treat-oriented holidays?

◆ How do we explain this to babysitters, day care people, and other caretakers?

◆ Why am I so angry?

◆ What do we do for birthday parties and other social occasions?

◆ How do I handle the well-meaning-but-cookie-slipping friends?

◆ My family is in denial—how do we explain this to them?

◆ Can we ever go out to dinner?

◆ How do we travel?

◆ Can I send my child to camp?

◆ What do I do when he cheats on his diet and intentionally eats gluten?

◆ What should we do if he accidentally gets gluten?

◆ Will he suffer from teasing and peer pressure?

◆ How do I help him handle this emotionally so he can be "just a kid"?

◆ Why doesn't my (insert family member) understand?

◆ Will he outgrow this?

◆ Can I ever shop at a "regular" grocery store again?

◆ Does the whole family need to adjust their diets too?

◆ How healthy is the gluten-free/casein-free diet?

◆ Will there be any nutritional deficiencies?

These are things that most *other* parents never need to give a second thought to. Things that consume those of us raising kids on a "special" diet, frustrate us, and cause us to feel anger, guilt, and sadness. They are, however, most definitely things that we can learn to deal with. This book will remind you that you're not alone, and that it does get easier. It's a compilation of lessons we've learned, most of them the hard way, and advice we've gathered over the years. I hope that you will find it helpful in raising *your* happy, healthy gluten-free/casein-free kids.

A Word about Terminology

This book is intended to be useful to parents of children who have any dietary restrictions, but, in particular, focuses on the gluten-free lifestyle.

There are many reasons people may put their kids on a gluten-free diet, including:

- ◆ Gluten intolerance/sensitivity (an inability to eat foods containing gluten). This includes children who have been diagnosed with or are suspected to have:
- ◆ celiac disease,
- ◆ gluten-sensitive enteropathy (GSE),
- ◆ nontropical sprue, and
- ◆ dermatitis herpetiformis

…which are all just different names for the same disorder. We refer to all of these conditions as gluten sensitivity or celiac disease throughout this book. We will also be talking about:

- ◆ autism spectrum disorders (including Asperger syndrome),
- ◆ ADD/ADHD,
- ◆ allergies,
- ◆ autoimmune diseases.

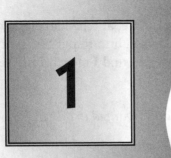

1

What It's Like to Be a Gluten-Free Kid

"I think about baseball, my friends, riding my motorcycle, and school. What I can or can't eat isn't really that big of a deal."

—Tyler Korn (at age 10)

Kids have such an awesome perspective on things. As parents, we worry that they'll feel "different," or "sad," or that they'll have a tough time with the gluten-free lifestyle and it will negatively affect their lives in some way, and later in this book I address those many emotions you may be feeling that are really quite normal.

But what I've found after many, many years of talking with gluten-free kids is that their perception is quite different from ours as adults, and especially ours as parents. For many kids, it's not the big deal that we parents make it.

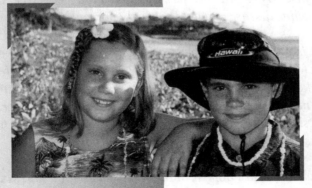

When Tyler was too young to really articulate his thoughts on the gluten-free lifestyle, I used to wish I could read his mind. I worried and wondered: Is this a big deal to you? Does it bother you? Are you okay with it? Obviously I wouldn't ask him those questions—it would have put doubt into his mind and made him wonder if he *should* have a problem with it.

By the time he was 11, though, Tyler was plenty articulate, and he had eight years of living a gluten-free lifestyle under his little belt. So I asked him to put his thoughts in writing about what it's like to be a kid with celiac disease, and I must admit his response was enlightening—and relieving:

Hello, my name is Tyler Korn. I'm eleven years old, and I wanted to talk about my experience with celiac disease.

When I was little, we didn't know what was wrong with me, but my parents knew I was really sick. Back then I was just eating regular food like you guys, and I would start getting sick. I don't remember it now, but my parents say that I was so sick they were scared I might even die. They took me to a bunch of doctors, and no one could figure out what was wrong. Finally we met a doctor who realized I was very sick, and he sent us to another doctor who figured out I had celiac disease.

Having celiac disease doesn't bother me. My friends all understand, and some of them even say they want their hamburgers without buns, or their ice cream in a bowl instead of a cone. We make a lot of our own breads and cookies and things, and I do a lot of cooking myself!

Really, it's not something I think about very often. I'm busy with baseball, motocross, and other sports, and it seems like those are the things I think about. My parents ask me sometimes what it feels like to have celiac disease, but it really doesn't feel like anything. It's really not that big of a deal. Maybe it used to be for them, but it isn't for me.

My parents asked me to write some advice for you parents who have kids with celiac disease. I guess my advice is: Don't freak out. It's probably really confusing and scary at first—I don't know, because I don't remember that part of it. But these days, it's just no big deal. I hope that makes you feel better...to know that we kids with celiac disease can lead perfectly normal lives.

The other advice I'd give is to let your kids be in control. I read my own labels and make all of my own food decisions. Sometimes my parents get scared that I'm going to make mistakes, but I know what I'm doing. (I am almost a man!) Sometimes I do make a mistake, and I get a really bad stomach ache—worse than the flu. It feels like a sharp pain in my stomach, and sometimes it makes me tired and lazy. But it goes away, and then I know not to eat that food again!

I hope you all enjoy this book, and I hope it makes it easier for you and your family to deal with celiac disease.

Good luck!

Mom's Postscript

Tyler isn't an 11-year-old kid any more (where does the time go?!?)—he's a young man in his 20s. I'd be lying if I said he has perfectly adhered to the gluten-free diet all these years. Much to my chagrin, he has cheated—and unfortunately, he doesn't feel the discomfort he used to feel when he eats gluten. I say that's unfortunate, because he no longer has that physical negative association with gluten that he had when he was younger. And considering that he is, in many ways, the "poster boy" for gluten-free kids, I've been sadly disappointed to find out about his choice to cheat.

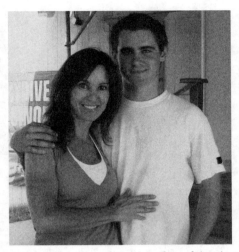

These days our conversations about cheating are higher level, reminding him in physiological detail of the damage he's doing to his body—and he is once again committed to being vigilant about his gluten-free lifestyle.

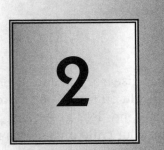

Should My Kid Be Gluten-Free?

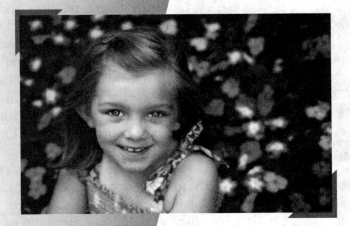

To be…or not to be…gluten-free. It's a big question, especially for parents when it concerns their child, because any parent knows we would spare our children pain, difficulty, or discomfort if we could. Some of you are considering cutting out gluten *and* casein, and there are common concerns: Will it affect her social life? Make it harder for her to fit in? Will it be "unnecessarily" difficult on her? Will it significantly improve her health or behavior? Is it really necessary? Good questions, but ones that can't be answered with simple answers.

There are many reasons to consider a gluten-free diet for your child. For some parents it's an option, and many variables should be considered. For others, the gluten-free diet is not an option, but a necessary step toward improving the health of their child.

Celiac Disease

If your child has been properly diagnosed with celiac disease, you don't need to waste much time pondering whether or not she should be gluten-free. The answer is yes. Unequivocally. No cheating, no occasional indulgences, no "let's give this a try." Although you don't have any choice about whether to put your child on a gluten-free diet, you *can* look forward to your child's improved health shortly after embarking upon the new lifestyle.

Celiac disease is a genetic disorder in which the ingestion of gluten triggers an autoimmune response that causes the body to destroy the lining of the small intestine. The specific area that gets destroyed is the same area responsible for absorbing iron, folic acid, fat-soluble vitamins, and other important nutrients. So until the body has healed (by being gluten-free), people are at risk for developing sometimes-serious nutritional deficiencies.

Occurring in approximately one percent of the population, celiac disease is the most common genetic disease of mankind, yet most people who have it are never diagnosed. Think about that—they have a chronic disease that may be causing all sorts of health

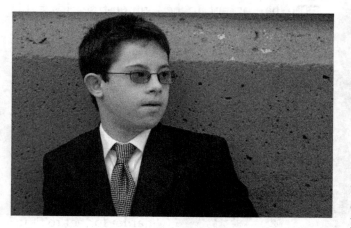

issues, and it could be fully controlled by diet alone! If someone is diagnosed, all first- and second-degree relatives should be tested, as their chances of having the condition are much higher than the general population.

Symptoms of celiac disease, which is sometimes referred to as sprue, are all over the board. A common misconception is that people with celiac disease all have diarrhea or other gastrointestinal disorders, when in reality, most do not. Symptoms can include irritability, headaches, fatigue, mood disorders, joint pain, and myriad others.

The beauty is that for people with celiac disease, no matter how mild or severe the symptoms, a gluten-free diet fully restores health. If your child was sick, irritable, or had behavioral issues, you'll likely see remarkable improvement after a very short time being gluten-free. See Chapter 22 for a detailed look at celiac disease.

Gluten Sensitivity/Gluten Intolerance

Defining gluten sensitivity is difficult, primarily because testing for any type of gluten sensitivity is squishy, at best. Where there are very specific and sensitive tests for celiac disease, testing for gluten sensitivity or intolerance that is not categorized as celiac disease is not well defined. Furthermore, many people are "diagnosed" as having gluten sensitivity when in fact they have celiac disease. Until there are better testing protocols, it's difficult to make a clear-cut distinction.

For the purposes of this book, we'll refer to gluten sensitivity the way most people do: a sensitivity or intolerance to gluten that is not clearly diagnosed as being celiac disease.

The good news is that, as is the case with celiac disease, a gluten-free diet fully restores health. The biggest question you'll face if your child has been "diagnosed" (it's in quotes because there's no great test yet) with gluten sensitivity is how strict do you have to be? With celiac disease, you need to be 100 percent strict about following the diet. With gluten sensitivity, it's not as clear-cut.

There is controversy about this, but in my opinion, you should be just as diligent about the gluten-free diet as if your child had been diagnosed with celiac disease. That means 100 percent. The reason I feel strongly about this is because the testing lines are blurred. What if it *is* celiac disease? What if the tests you got aren't as conclusive as you assume, and your child actually does have celiac disease? You could be doing her great harm by allowing her the occasional gluten indulgence, and it's just not worth it.

Autism, ADD, ADHD

Autism spectrum disorders (ASD), Attention Deficit Disorder (ADD), and Attention-Deficit/Hyperactivity Disorder (ADHD) sometimes respond well to a gluten-free (and casein-free) diet.

If you're putting your child on a gluten-free diet—or considering doing so—for this reason, I commend you and encourage you to do so with diligence. Admittedly, cutting gluten, casein, and sometimes soy as well out of a child's diet isn't easy. The difficulties are compounded if you're dealing with a child with ASD. First, he or she may experience food "jags" (an insistence on eating the same food meal after meal—common in people with autism). Second, your child may also be physiologically addicted to the very foods you're trying to eliminate (see Chapter 23 for why this may be).

But going gluten free may be worth it—very worth it—if your child experiences the benefits that have been widely reported.

Well-done scientific, double-blind, placebo-controlled studies to examine the effects of a gluten-free/casein-free diet on kids on the autism spectrum are sparse, but underway. Details of the mechanisms involved are fascinating, and covered in detail in Chapter 23.

Wheat Allergies

If your child has an allergy to wheat, she needs to be essentially—but not thoroughly—gluten-free. That is, she can't eat wheat, but she can eat barley (a component of gluten, which means it's off-limits on a gluten-free diet) and rye (another component of gluten). For more details on exactly what gluten is, see Chapter 3.

But before you consider your child to have wheat allergies, read on. Lots of people *think* they have wheat allergies when they don't.

There are specific tests for wheat allergies, the most common of which include elimination diet, food challenges, skin test, and blood test.

- ◆ **Elimination diet:** In this test, the suspected allergen—in this case wheat—is removed from the diet. Gradually, under a doctor's supervision, foods are added back into the diet to see if symptoms return.
- ◆ **Food challenge:** This test, again, must be done under the careful supervision of a doctor, and is often done at a hospital. For this challenge, you eat small amounts of wheat, gradually increasing the amount you eat, while being monitored for allergic reactions.

Keep in mind that diagnosing someone with a wheat allergy is easier if the person has the same reaction every time they eat wheat-containing food. But usually people eat foods in combination, so it's tough to distinguish which food is causing the problem. That's why a skin or blood test may provide a more conclusive diagnosis.

- ◆ **Skin test:** Tiny drops of purified extracts of wheat proteins are pricked onto your skin's surface, usually on your back or forearm. After 15 minutes, the doctor or nurse checks for signs of allergic reaction. If there is one, it will be a red, itchy bump that will disappear within half an hour or so.
- ◆ **Blood test:** The blood test looks for specific antibodies to the protein fragments in wheat.

Symptoms of a wheat allergy are vast. Some people have a skin reaction such as hives or swelling. Others have respiratory reactions such as asthma or allergic rhinitis. Severe reactions are called anaphylaxis, and can be life-threatening—the airway constricts or heart rhythm may become altered, resulting in complete airway obstruction, shock, or even death.

In many cases, though, the symptom of wheat allergy is mild-to-severe gastrointestinal distress—the same symptom seen in gluten sensitivity and celiac disease.

That's why some people *think* they have wheat allergies, but in fact they don't. The first two types of tests to detect wheat allergies described in this section are common ways of determining whether someone has an allergy or not, yet they don't distinguish between an *allergic* reaction and something else. Often people are told (or assume) they have wheat allergies, when in fact they have gluten sensitivity or celiac disease.

Gluten Allergies

There's no such thing. There are allergies to the things that comprise gluten (wheat, rye, and barley)—but gluten is the umbrella term for those foods (for a more technical definition of gluten, see Chapter 3), and people don't have an allergy to gluten, per se. Saying you have an allergy to gluten is like saying you have an allergy to food. You may have allergies to *some* foods, but not to food itself.

Autoimmune Diseases

While there is little hard-core scientific evidence to support the claims, many people believe that the symptoms of autoimmune diseases (other than celiac disease) improve on a gluten-free diet. Examples of these autoimmune conditions include multiple sclerosis, lupus, and fibromyalgia.

Many autoimmune diseases have symptoms that mimic those of celiac disease, such as chronic pain, fatigue, and gastrointestinal distress.

In some people whose symptoms for a non-celiac disease improve on a gluten-free diet, it's likely that in addition to the disease they've been diagnosed with, they have celiac disease or gluten intolerance. Others may actually be misdiagnosed as having another condition when they actually have celiac disease or gluten sensitivity. And others may truly find relief for their non-celiac autoimmune disease on a gluten-free diet for a variety of reasons (see more detail in Chapter 22).

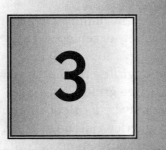

3

Gluten-Free/ Casein-Free: The Ground Rules of the Diet

"I'd like to try a gluten-free casein-free diet for my child, but I have no idea where to start. It seems like there's nothing he can eat."

—Deborah H.

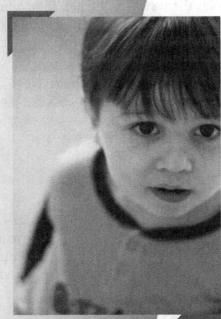

If you're considering a gluten-free and possibly casein-free diet for your child, the first thing you'll need to do is figure out what he can eat! Although the diet may seem overwhelming and restrictive, the good news is that the list of things he *can* eat is a lot longer than the list of things he can't. Until you're sure about a food or ingredient, you'll need to stick to this fundamental rule: **When in doubt, leave it out.**

In this chapter we'll take a look at the basics of the gluten-free and casein-free diets. Later in the book we'll apply those basics to everyday living, with meal and snack ideas, as well as shopping, cooking, and preparation tips.

What Is Gluten?

So what *is* gluten, anyway? You would think it would be an easy question to answer—but it's not easy—and that's partly because there's a lot of incorrect information floating around about what contains gluten and what doesn't. It's also because there are different definitions of gluten. Most are not technically correct, yet those are the ones widely accepted. So let's start by taking a look at the different definitions of gluten.

The common-but-technically-incorrect definition of gluten is: Gluten is a protein found in wheat, rye, barley, and derivatives of these three grains.

Oats in and of themselves are gluten-free, yet there may be a risk of contamination from wheat, rye, or barley, so oats are avoided on a strict gluten-free diet. The exception is if you can find certified gluten-free oats. (See more about oats and the gluten-free certification process later in this chapter.)

The not-so-common-but-technically-correct definition of gluten: For those who are interested, I'll give you the technically correct definition of gluten, but you have to promise to read the history behind it, lest you be tempted to e-mail me and tell me I'm all wrong.

Historically, gluten comes from wheat and only wheat (please don't e-mail me and say I'm wrong—read on!). Gluten is what food and grain scientists refer to as a "storage protein." Over time, the word gluten became a general term for "prolamins," a peptide sequence (protein fraction) found in lots of different grains. The prolamins that cause damage to people with gluten sensitivity, celiac disease, and the related conditions we discuss in this book are found in wheat (gliadin), rye (secalin), and barley (hordein). But other grains have prolamins, too. Corn's prolamin is called zein. Rice's is called orzenin. But their prolamins aren't toxic to people with gluten sensitivity and celiac disease.

So if gluten comes from wheat and only wheat, how did they all get lumped together? At some point, doctors made an association between wheat and celiac disease. It became widely accepted that gluten makes them sick, and when they realized that rye and barley made them sick too, the conclusion was that rye and barley must have gluten. It was a sideways conclusion that wasn't quite right, but time marches on, and the definition has stuck.

> For the purposes of this book, we'll accept the technically incorrect but common definition of gluten: gluten is a protein found in wheat, rye, and barley.

Oats Notes

Many of you must be wondering, "but what about oats?!" Yep, lots of people wonder, because there's so much conflicting information out there, and because it's not an easy question to answer. Technically, oats don't have that offending prolamin portion we discussed in the previous section. So technically, they're gluten-free, and not harmful to people avoiding gluten.

But during the farming, cultivation, storage, and manufacturing process, there are many opportunities for oats to become contaminated with wheat and other gluten-containing grains, thereby making them off-limits to those on a strict GF diet.

There are, however, oats that are certified gluten-free and safe even for those on the strictest of diets. They're grown on farmland dedicated only to oats and other gluten-free grains, processed and manufactured in gluten-free facilities, and certified as gluten-free. (There are a couple of certification programs—read more about those in the sidebar on page 18.) You can find these certified GF oats online, at natural foods stores that carry GF items, or in the specialty sections that carry GF items in your grocery stores.

Gluten-Free at a Glance

Gluten can be hidden in a lot of things, so you'll need to learn to read labels carefully. The reason it's not so straightforward is because there are "derivatives" of gluten-containing grains that may contain gluten. Those are listed in the safe and forbidden ingredients list in the Appendix, and are usually found in additives and flavorings.

The simple list of grains not allowed on the gluten-free diet is:
◆ Wheat
◆ Rye
◆ Barley
◆ Oats (see the section on oats earlier in this chapter)
◆ Triticale (a hybrid of wheat and rye)

At the risk of overstating the obvious, you need to avoid pretty much anything with the word wheat in it. This includes hydrolyzed wheat protein, wheat starch, wheat germ, and so on. Wheat *grass* is an exception (see the sidebar that follows).

But it gets a little tricky, because there are several names for and types of wheat. Watch out for:
◆ bulgur,
◆ cake flour,
◆ couscous,
◆ durum (also spelled duram),
◆ einkorn,
◆ farina,
◆ flour,
◆ frumento,
◆ graham,
◆ kamut,
◆ matzoh, matzah, matzo,
◆ semolina,
◆ spelt, and
◆ seitan.

In case you missed it in the list above, you need to avoid **spelt**. It's so commonly sold as a "wheat alternative," that it deserves a second mention here—spelt *is* wheat and while it may be sold as a "wheat alternative" (I'm not sure how they get away with that!), it is absolutely *not* allowed on a gluten-free diet.

Sorting Out Grasses, Berries, and Germ...

Wheat grass, like all grasses, is safe on the gluten-free diet! I know it's confusing because I just finished saying almost anything with "wheat" in it is off-limits. But grass hasn't sprouted and formed the gluten-containing peptides that cause problems in people who need to strictly avoid gluten. Sprouted grains, however, should be avoided because you don't know where in the sprouting process the grain is. It could be okay, but it might not.

Berries (e.g., wheat berries) are definitely not safe, because they're the seed kernels and definitely contain the toxic portion of the protein. There's some debate about bran (as in wheat bran), so until research is done to confirm it one way or the other, you should stick by the rule of thumb: when in doubt, leave it out.

Grains and Starches Allowed on the Gluten-free Diet

What people tend to miss most on the gluten-free diet is that starchy, fill-you-up feeling that wheat provides. Miss it no more! There are plenty of gluten-free grains and starches, some of which are far more nutritious than wheat ever wished it could be. They include:

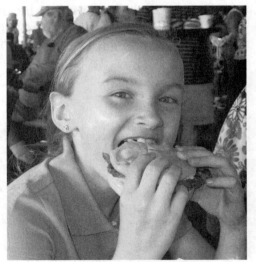

- ◆ amaranth
- ◆ arrowroot
- ◆ beans
- ◆ buckwheat/groats/kasha
- ◆ chickpea (garbanzo, besan, cici, chana, or gram—not to be confused with graham, which *does* have gluten)
- ◆ corn
- ◆ garfava
- ◆ Job's tears
- ◆ mesquite (pinole)
- ◆ millet
- ◆ Montina® (Indian ricegrass)
- ◆ oats (gluten-free, but they may be contaminated with wheat and other grains)
- ◆ potato

- quinoa (hie)
- ragi
- rice
- sorghum
- soy
- tapioca (gari, cassava, casaba, manioc, yucca)
- taro root
- teff

Glutinous Rice

Glutinous rice sounds like it has gluten in it, but it doesn't! Also called sweet rice or mocha, glutinous rice is made from extra high-starch short-grain rice. You'll find it in Asian dishes like sushi, but it is also used to thicken sauces and desserts.

Foods That Are Usually Gluten-free

In general, these foods are usually gluten-free (these refer to plain, unseasoned foods without additives and processed products):

- meat
- poultry
- fish
- seafood
- fruits
- vegetables
- nuts
- legumes
- beans
- berries
- eggs
- dairy products

Gums

Gums such as xanthan gum and guar gum are gluten-free! You'll find they're called for frequently when making gluten-free baked goods, because they help to give that spongy, elastic texture that wheat flour usually provides. Careful, though. For some people these gums can have a laxative effect, which is sometimes mistakenly confused as a reaction to gluten.

Avoiding Hidden Sources of Gluten

Some ingredients listed on labels *may* contain gluten—or they may not. It depends upon the source of the ingredient in question. For instance, modified food starch may be derived from corn, in which case it is okay, or from wheat, in which case it is, of course, not gluten-free.

Foods That Usually Contain Gluten

There are lots of foods that you have to assume have gluten in them. Of course, there are special gluten-free varieties of these foods, but unless you're buying specialty products, you can assume the following foods will usually have gluten in them:

- beer
- bread, bread crumbs, biscuits
- cereal

- communion wafers
- cornbread
- croutons
- cookies, cakes, cupcakes, doughnuts, muffins, pastries, pie crusts, brownies, and other baked goods
- crackers
- gravies, sauces, and roux
- imitation seafood (e.g., crab)
- licorice
- marinades such as teriyaki
- pasta
- pizza crust
- pretzels
- soy sauce
- stuffing

Play Doh

Watch out for Play Doh! It has gluten (wheat) in it. But in Chapter 16 I give you a recipe for making your own GF play dough. You can also find gluten-free varieties sold online.

Alternative Grains Are Gluten-Free

I'm a big fan of alternative "grains." I put "grains" in quotation marks because most of them aren't actually grains at all—many are seeds or flowers. But they're ultra nutritious, delicious, and gluten-free, and I encourage you to add them to your meal plans. Here are some of the nutritional powerhouses:

- **Amaranth**—Loaded with fiber, iron, calcium, and other vitamins and minerals, amaranth is also high in the amino acids lysine, methionine, and cysteine, and is an excellent source of protein.
- **Arrowroot**—An easily digested and nutritious starch, arrowroot is a fine white powder with a look and texture similar to cornstarch. The translucent paste has no flavor, and will set to an almost clear gel. (Careful: the arrowroot *biscuits* made for babies usually have wheat flour added to them so they're not gluten-free.)
- **Buckwheat** (soba)—The name would lead you to believe there's wheat in buckwheat, but there's not. It's not even related to wheat, and, in fact, isn't even a true cereal grain. It's a fruit and is a distant cousin of garden-variety rhubarb. Buckwheat is super high in protein and many of the B vitamins, as well as the minerals phosphorus, magnesium, iron, copper, manganese, and zinc.
- **Mesquite** (pinole)—Yep, it's the same stuff you might throw on the grill to make foods taste smoky and sweet. Mesquite flour is a low-glycemic-index flour (it's a 25, for those of you who care), helpful in controlling blood sugar levels. Furthermore, soluble fibers such as galactomannin gum in the seeds and pods slow absorption of nutrients, which also help in controlling blood sugar levels.

◆ **Millet**—Millet is packed with vitamins, minerals, phytochemicals, and other nutrients. High in iron, magnesium, phosphorus, and potassium, it is also loaded with fiber and protein, as well as the B-complex vitamins, including niacin, thiamin, and riboflavin. Millet is more nutritious than many traditional grains, and is very easy to digest.

◆ **Montina** (Indian Ricegrass)—Montina® is actually a trademarked name for Indian ricegrass produced by a company called Amazing Grains. Much like *Kleenex* has become interchangeable for the word *tissue,* Montina is becoming the more common name for Indian ricegrass. It has a bold flavor, and is loaded with fiber and protein.

◆ **Quinoa** (hie)—pronounced "KEEN-wa" and also called *hie,* pronounced "HE-uh," quinoa is yet another of the "grains" that isn't really a grain—it's actually a seed packed with lysine and other amino acids that make it a complete protein. It's also high in phosphorus, calcium, iron, vitamin E, and assorted B vitamins, as well as fiber.

◆ **Sorghum** (milo, jowar, jowari, cholam)—Sorghum is another of the oldest known grains (that isn't a true cereal grain), and has been a major source of nutrition in Africa and India for centuries. Now also grown in the United States, sorghum is generating excitement as a gluten-free insoluble fiber, and is probably best known for the syrup made from one of its varieties.

◆ **Teff** (tef)—Small package; big nutrition. Teff is the smallest of the grains-that-aren't-true-cereal-grains, and in fact the name itself means "lost," because if you drop it on the ground, you probably won't find it. A staple grain in Ethiopia for nearly 5,000 years, teff packs a protein content of nearly 12 percent, and is five times richer in calcium, iron, and potassium than any other grain.

For years there have been rumors that some of these "alternative grains" aren't safe for people with gluten sensitivity or celiac disease. They *are,* in fact, gluten-free. Some people may have had reactions to these grains (as they would to corn, soy, or other allergens or foods to which they may have a sensitivity), but it's not a gluten reaction.

Remember the fundamental rule: Regardless of whether or not a food contains gluten, if it makes you sick, don't eat it!

Putting an End to the Controversy

If you've been researching the gluten-free diet on your own, you most likely have found lots of conflicting information. Some sources will say, for instance, that vinegar has gluten—others will say it doesn't. Well, I'm here to help put an end to the controversy.

Once thought to be off-limits or questionable, the following ingredients are no longer on the "we're not sure" list. All of them are safe for people on a strict gluten-free diet! (The gluten-free status of these ingredients applies to ingredients produced in North America. Other countries may have different manufacturing processes.)

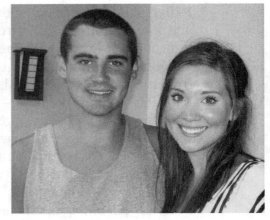

- caramel color
- modified food starch
- wheat grass
- vinegar (except malt vinegar, which is off limits)
- maltodextrin (except in pharmaceuticals)
- citric acid
- hydrolyzed vegetable protein (HVP)
- hydrolyzed plant protein (HPP)
- alcohol (distilled)
- mono and diglycerides
- vanilla and vanilla extract
- flavoring extracts
- yeast (except brewer's yeast, which does contain gluten)
- citric acid
- starch (except in pharmaceuticals)
- dextrin

Gluten-free Certification Makes It Easy to Know for Sure

There are a couple of certification programs that have easy-to-recognize logos so you can see at a glance that an item has been certified as being gluten-free. The first certification program was launched by the Gluten Intolerance Group (GIG) and is called the Gluten-Free Certification Organization (GFCO). GFCO has a logo that says "Certified Gluten-Free," and it indicates that a food contains less than 10 ppm (parts per million) of gluten—a level far below the widely accepted safe limit of 20 ppm. The GFCO checks the ingredient lists, tests foods, and even inspects the manufacturing plants to ensure that the food has gluten-free ingredients and that there is no contamination in the production process.

Celiac Sprue Association (CSA) also has a certification with a seal indicating that products are gluten-free (including oat-free) with less than 5 ppm of gluten. Both of these logos make it easy to spot a food that is assured to be safe on the gluten-free diet.

Contamination

Most of the controversy about the gluten-free status of certain foods revolves around the issue of contamination. Is the food product that appears to be gluten-free actually contaminated in some way with gluten?

Contamination can occur in otherwise GF food items in a variety of ways:

> *"My brother did some research on celiac disease and said that we shouldn't let our son eat the fries at McDonald's because they might be fried in the same oil as something with gluten in it. Do I really need to be concerned about how the food is cooked?"*
>
> —Leanna W.

- ◆ **Preparation:** Gluten-free foods are prepared with the same utensils, on the same cooking surfaces, or in the same "medium" (such as oil) as gluten-containing foods.
- ◆ **Processing:** When commercial products are processed, they are generally on what is referred to as a "line," which is usually a type of conveyor belt that physically moves the product through its production cycle. Sometimes a gluten-containing product is processed on the line right next to a gluten-free product. Other times, the same line is used for both types of products. While at first this may seem as though it would obviously turn a gluten-free product into a celiac response waiting to happen, it's important to note that the Food and Drug Administration requires all food manufacturers and ingredient suppliers to follow careful guidelines called Good Manufacturing Practices (GMP) when cleaning equipment.
- ◆ **Bulk Bins:** The bulk bins at grocery stores can be contaminated because they sit close to one another, and people may dig into several different bins with the same scoop.
- ◆ **Growing Grains:** Sometimes gluten-free grains will be grown in fields close to gluten-containing grains. Some people believe that cross-contamination can occur while the plants are still growing.

So, how seriously do you take the issue of contamination? I'm not touching that one with a ten-foot pole. It's a personal decision that boils down to: How crazy do you want to make yourself?

Of course, you need to be aware of the possibility of contamination, and make wise food choices. If you're at a fast food restaurant and they have the fries cooking in the same oil as the onion rings, you might want to think twice about those fries. Not that the oil itself would *necessarily* cause a problem, but surely there are pieces of the onion-ring breading floating around, and it's pretty likely that they could make their way into your fry basket.

How Perfect Do We Have to Be?

Allow me to make a subtle but important distinction here. Being diligent about the diet, especially if your child has celiac disease or a severe intolerance, is not an option. The question here is how stringent you need to be in figuring out whether a food is gluten-free or not. It's yet another controversial subject, with vocal and knowledgeable advocates at both ends of the spectrum. Of course, without a doubt, you should be as diligent about keeping your child as gluten-free as possible.

> *"By the time we've considered the possibility of cross-contamination, whether or not distillation actually eliminates any trace of gluten, and how foods are processed, it seems like there's nothing left that we can feed our daughter. How perfect do we have to be?"*
>
> —*Ted D.*

Having said that, no one is perfect. Don't expect yourself to be, and certainly don't expect your child to be. Don't beat yourself or your child up over the mistakes that will be made.

One of the most positive, constructive approaches I've heard comes from Ann Whelan, editor and publisher of the *Gluten-Free Living* magazine and a person with celiac disease herself. The following is an excerpt from an editorial she published in the March/April 1999 edition:

"Let's stop worrying that the next potential trace of possible gluten that might find its way into our bodies is going to kill us. Unscientific exaggerations like this scare and mislead people, make them depressed and even cause many to cheat on the grounds that it makes no difference since we all live in a gluten-filled world and are likely doomed anyway.

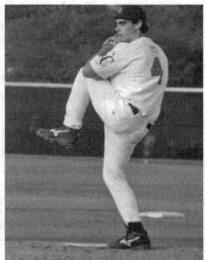

"Yes, we all need to stay as gluten-free as possible, but responsibly gluten-free. Fearing a scientifically unmeasurable, theoretically impossible but not proven-beyond-a-skeptical-celiac-doubt molecule of gliadin has an unhealthful paranoid tone to it. It's a bit like deciding to stay indoors in the dark when the sun is up once the words basal cell cancer enter your life."

Thinking Outside the Food Box

It's not just food you need to think about when you're avoiding gluten. Everything you ingest—including medications and some other products—can cause problems if it's not gluten-free.

Medications and Supplements

You know how it is with kids. They wait until doctors' offices are closed for the weekend or you're headed out of town before they cautiously mumble, "I'm not feeling good." Feel their forehead, and sure enough—hot and sweaty, and the cough is starting already.

No problem, right? A little cough syrup and fever-reducer, and . . . uh oh. Is it gluten-free? Well, 2 a.m. on a Saturday isn't the time to realize you have no idea which medications are gluten-free. Many contain starch (which is okay in foods, but not necessarily pharmaceuticals), fillers, stabilizers, flavorings, or other ingredients that could contain gluten.

Do your homework in advance. If there are medications your child takes frequently, be sure to find out which brands are okay. For prescription medications, a pharmacist can help you use a Physician's Desk Reference (PDR) to look up ingredients. You may need to take it a step farther and call the drug manufacturer to know for sure. (There's more in the next chapter about calling manufacturers.)

Helpful Idea! If your pharmacist helps you determine which medications are gluten-free, have him or her make a note of gluten-free medications in his or her records. Not only will this be useful for you in the future, but it will help others who may inquire as well.

Over-the-counter medications always have a toll-free number on the label. You should call that number and inquire whether the exact product you're using is gluten-free. And remember, products change! Just because it's okay today doesn't mean that same product will be okay tomorrow.

Another Helpful Tip: Once you've determined that a medication is safe, write "GF" in permanent marker on the package. That way you won't be questioning yourself in the middle of the night when you're wondering if the medication is safe or not.

Bringing It Out of the Bathroom

There are lots of questions about whether or not you need to avoid bathroom items such as lotion, shampoos, and toothpaste. The answers, as always, aren't exactly straightforward, but let's take a look at what you need to be aware of.

Shampoos: I have become so accustomed to reading labels that I find myself reading ingredients on nonfood items. It was in the shower that I realized that nearly every shampoo we use contains wheat! Many people have asked whether this can cause a reaction in someone with celiac disease. In other words, can gluten be absorbed through the skin? The answer is no, according to John Zone, M.D., a dermatologist who is an expert on dermatitis herpetiformis (DH)—a sister condition to celiac disease that manifests itself on the skin (see more about DH in Chapter 22). Dr. Zone says that gluten that is present in topically applied make-ups and lotions is not absorbed, because the protein molecules in gluten are too large. So shampoos are fine, as long as you don't eat them.

Lotions: Theoretically, if you're not eating your lotion, you're okay. But think about how you prepare food. Do you have lotion on your hands that could get onto the food you're eating? Do you lick your fingers when you eat? Do your fingers get in your kid's mouth when you feed him? Those are the things to watch for as far as lotions are concerned

Toothpaste: Toothpaste is supposed to be used in miniscule amounts, and of course, you're supposed to spit it out. But kids often smear a gob of toothpaste the size of a Tootsie Roll on their toothbrush, and if it tastes good enough, they'll swallow it and go for seconds. Most toothpastes are gluten free, but it's a good idea to check with the manufacturer to make sure there aren't any hidden sources of gluten.

Lipstick and Other Types of Make-up: You're probably not taking big bites out of your lipstick, but you probably do lick your lips. And if you kiss . . . that lipstick ends up on the lips of the other person. That's when it can present a problem. Other types of make-up, including foundation, mascara, and eye shadow won't present a problem, whether or not they are gluten free.

Pet Food

When you're taking inventory of your gluten-free zones, don't forget about the pet food. Most dog and cat foods are loaded with gluten. What does that have to do with your kids? Well, more than just a few of them have been known to finagle Fido's food from time to time. The dry kind, of course. If yours are prone to pilfering from your pets, you should definitely nip that in the bud.

Safe and Forbidden Ingredients

A comprehensive list of safe and forbidden ingredients for people on the gluten-free diet is included in the Appendix at the back of this book. This list, also available online at www.celiac.com, was compiled by Scott Adams. It's a good idea to make or print out a copy of this list, and then keep it posted in a kitchen cabinet, or where you can easily access it when you need to.

Casein-Free at a Glance

Many of you are eliminating casein from your child's diet as well as gluten. Like gluten, casein is a protein—but instead of being found in grains, casein is found in milk products (milk from any mammal). The main sources of casein include:

◆ Milk
◆ Whey
◆ Cheese
◆ Yogurt
◆ Cream
◆ Butter
◆ Ice cream

That's the short list of foods containing casein. Unfortunately, like gluten, casein is found in lots of foods in various forms. It's an emulsifier and binding agent in foods such as vegetarian "cheese," vegetarian "meats," cereals, breads, and supplements. You should also watch for casein in:

- ◆ Soups
- ◆ Sauces/Dressings
- ◆ Snack foods
- ◆ Bread and anything in breadcrumbs
- ◆ Nutrition Bars
- ◆ Protein Shakes

The good news is that casein is usually easy to spot on a label. Look for ingredients including milk (which must be called out specifically on the label), whey, and anything with the word "casein" in it (such as caseinate).

Labeling Law Helps in Avoiding Wheat and Milk

A law enacted in the United States in 2006 has made life much easier for those of us avoiding gluten and/or casein. Called the Food Allergen Labeling and Consumer Protection Act (FALCPA), this law mandates that food labels must clearly indicate if a food contains wheat or milk. (Labels must also indicate if a food contains eggs, fish, shellfish, tree nuts, peanuts, and soybeans.)

This helps immensely, but remember that wheat-free doesn't mean gluten-free. A food can, for instance, contain malt (from barley) or rye, making it wheat-free but not gluten-free.

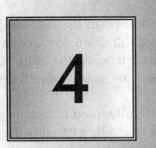

Helpful Hints for the Newbie

"We're just getting started with the diet. We're looking for ANY tips that would make it easier."

—Dan and Debbie F.

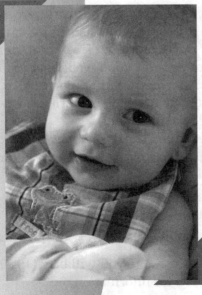

I was a newbie once. When Tyler was first diagnosed with celiac disease, our doctor, trying to be upbeat, nonchalantly explained that this would mean that we would just need to modify Ty's diet, and that we would need to eliminate—you may want to write this down, he suggested—wheat, oats, rye, and barley, which we're all supposed to know is what they use to make malt. Oh, and anything else that may contain gluten.

Hmmm. That really didn't sound too tough. After all, we were well-educated people—how hard could it be to cut out five ingredients? As I checked out of the doctor's office, they suggested I see the hospital dietitian, who had a list of gluten-free foods and forbidden ingredients. I figured it wouldn't hurt to have a little help, so I dropped by, figuring I would surely be her forty-third celiac mom that month, and asked her for the gluten-free foods list.

The five seconds it took her to register my request in her brain should have been my first clue that the folks at the hospital didn't come across this often. My second clue should have been that she had to dig through several folders before she finally pulled out a well-worn and obviously long-forgotten blue sheet that said, "Gluten-Free—Forbidden Ingredients."

I nearly choked when I saw the size-four font that literally filled the entire page with things my son could *not* have! There was even a back side! What happened to just wheat, oats, rye, barley and malt? "Oh," she explained, "gluten is in all sorts of ingredients you wouldn't normally think of," and she started to read to me off the sheet. I grumpily snatched it away from her. I can read myself, thank you very much.

That was in 1991, before anyone could just log onto the Internet and search for the information they needed. There were no books—no support groups that I knew of—I was truly all alone. I know what it's like to be a newbie.

Time's a tickin', Newbie. You need to dive right in. Kids need to eat, ya know! There are several things you can do right away that will help you take control and move forward. Knowledge is power, and the more you know, the more comfortable you'll feel.

In this chapter, I talk about some big-picture steps you'll want to take to get you off and running. Beyond the big-picture stuff, tips for daily living will be scattered throughout the other chapters in this book, such as the chapters that cover cooking and shopping.

Do Your Homework

Take some time to review this book and peruse the Internet, bookstores, and libraries for information on celiac disease, gluten sensitivity, autism, or whatever condition(s) your child has. The diet is one thing, but it's important to understand the medical condition, as well. There are several good websites with current research, product information, and resources. Having said that, don't believe everything you read. Websites are sprouting up faster than weeds in April, and "weeding" through websites to sort fact from fiction can be a nightmare.

With the popularity of the gluten-free diet soaring, books and articles are proliferating. They too are a mix of fact and fiction, so make sure the author is a trusted and respected authority on the subject.

Get Organized

There is *a lot* of information to digest, and you will be well-served to stay organized. Start a binder or file with sections for information on:
   ◆ gluten-free foods
   ◆ manufacturers' contact information and correspondence

- correspondence with restaurants
- resources (mail order food companies, for instance)
- organizations

See Chapter 12 for more information on collecting and organizing information.

Contact Support Groups

I'm not usually a "support group" type of person; I tend to want to dive in and figure things out on my own. But it's a good idea to reach out and find a local support group to see what they have to offer. (I also think they do wonderful work and choose to support them with time and finances, even though I don't imbibe myself.) There are all kinds of support groups—from more general groups for all kids on a gluten-free diet (like R.O.C.K.), to ones that are specific to your child's condition (e.g., autism). You might find something that resonates—or you might not. At a minimum, the group can probably offer you important information that will help you get started with the diet.

Local chapters of support groups hold regular meetings that you may wish to attend. For some parents, the value of these meetings is in finding that their child is not alone in their condition. Many parents enjoy the meetings because they feature knowledgeable speakers or take pleasure in the camaraderie of socializing with other families in the same boat. Others, frankly, don't enjoy the experience of a support group. If support groups aren't for you, that's fine; at least you know what they can offer if you choose to participate.

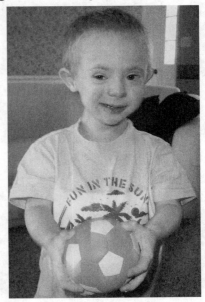

The Internet also offers opportunities for joining support groups and sharing information. In addition to websites that offer a myriad of information and services, there are groups called "Listservs"— these groups are basically a way to communicate by e-mail with others who have the same condition(s) your child has. They provide a forum for free postings to an e-mail list so you can see other people's posts and they can see yours. A good starting point for locating listservs is to visit the Yahoo! Groups website (http://groups.yahoo.com) and type "gluten free" into the box labeled "Find a Yahoo Group." You can share information, ask questions, and voice opinions.

Remember, though, the people submitting information to the LISTSERV—or to websites, for that matter—are not necessarily experts. Some of the information must be taken with a grain (gluten-free, of course) of salt.

Don't Be Afraid to Dive in and Feed Your Kid

True, the list of foods your child has to avoid for life is very long. But there is a much longer list of foods that your child *can* eat without a problem.

First, check out the lists of safe and forbidden foods in the Appendix and head to the grocery store to stock up on products that your child likes. Also, try out some of the gluten-free staples such as bread, pasta, and mixes for baked goods that are available from specialty sections of your grocery store, natural foods stores, and by phone or Internet. Then turn to the "Quick Meal Ideas" in Chapter 13. Here you will find more than enough tasty options for meals and snacks to keep your child happily fed until you feel knowledgeable enough to confidently plan your own menus again.

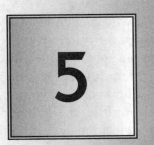

5

Panic, Anger, Grief, Denial, and Other Emotions You Can Look Forward To

"Every now and then I get really angry. I'm angry at rude people who treat Jake differently, I'm angry at my family and friends because they don't understand, I'm angry at God, I'm angry because there aren't more foods he can eat. When I get tired of being angry, I get sad and depressed. Will I always feel this way?"

—Terri W.

"No one seems to understand. I'm terrified to feed my own child! The diet seems so complicated, and the doctors made me feel like I could do great harm to my daughter if I make one mistake. I'm panicked to the point of not being able to think straight."

—Laura R.

"I feel like those parents who just have to cut gluten out of their kid's diet have it made. Gluten AND casein is really tough! I'm feeling so sorry for myself, and I hate myself for that."

—Ron W.

The Bittersweet Diagnosis... Then Panic Sets In

Ah, but it's a bittersweet diagnosis, isn't it? After a long ordeal, you're assured that your child will not need medication or surgery, and has a prognosis of perfect health. It's just that at first it seems there's nothing on the planet that you can feed him.

Most likely, you had a difficult time arriving at a diagnosis or a dietary intervention for your child. It's an all-too-common story. Your child is sick and getting sicker or has behavioral issues, yet doctors can't seem to figure out what's wrong.

Often they wave you away with some vague "explanation" of why your child has symptoms, but with no diagnosis and no understanding of how to make your kid feel better.

Those of us who know the symptoms of celiac disease can spot it a mile away, yet many doctors don't think of it, and some even refuse to test for it when it is suggested as a possibility. Doctors and nurses toss out possible explanations for your child's symptoms as though they're reviewing a grocery list: cystic fibrosis, check; blood disease, check; cancer, check. It's impossible to describe the sensations we experience while waiting to find out what's wrong with our babies.

People whose children have behavioral issues often have a long road to diagnosis, as well. Dismissed with platitudes like "he'll outgrow it" or "that's just his personality" do little but frustrate parents and waste precious time that could have at least provided answers and the hope of the possibility of dietary intervention.

No matter what the condition, the truth is that we really should be thankful once the diagnosis is made. In many children, the diagnosis is missed, and they suffer their entire lives with compromised health or unexplained behavioral issues. Others are misdiagnosed, and gluten continues to wreak havoc on their system, while the blame is erroneously placed on lactose intolerance, irritable bowel syndrome, or other conditions.

So, if your child has been diagnosed with celiac disease, gluten sensitivity, autism, or another condition that may improve on a gluten-free diet, you're fortunate. I know, it's hard to see beyond the "difficult" diet at first, but it does get easier, and there are many resources available to get you through it. A gluten-free lifestyle can be extremely healthy, and there are no medications required, no surgeries, and no long-term difficulties, if a strict GF diet is adhered to. Best of all, no matter what your child's issues, chances are good to great that he'll improve on a GF diet.

Riding the Emotional Roller Coaster

It's important to know that it's perfectly normal to experience a myriad of emotions when your child has been diagnosed with any condition, especially one that has a profound effect on your lifestyle. You're not selfish if you feel self-pity; you're not a "bad parent" if you find yourself angry; you're not alone if you feel an overwhelming sense of grief, and even loss.

"I'm so grief-stricken that I can't get beyond the questions whirling in my head: Will she feel 'different' on the diet? Will she be healthy? Will she be sad? How will she ever be able to go away to college?"

—Cherita T.

Many parents, while in the chasm of these sometimes-overwhelming emotions, withdraw and are unsure of what to do next. Understanding that these feelings are normal is an important step in overcoming them.

People tend to progress through a series of emotions in response to bad news or a loss. If you think about it, having your child diagnosed with a chronic disease or lifelong disability is a loss of a kind. Perhaps it is the loss of the image you may have had for your child's future. The specific meaning of this information varies widely among individuals. However, this type of event typically requires that people go through a period of adjustment in order to integrate the new information into their existing mental framework. Below is my take, as a parent who has not only been-there-done-that, but who has talked to literally thousands of other parents, on the adjustment process.

Panic

Generally, the first emotion you'll experience is *panic*. What on earth will you feed this child? What if you poison him? How do you explain the diet—the condition—to your friends and family? There are a number of issues that may be concerning you at this point, and they all must be sorted through before you can move on. It can feel quite overwhelming as implications and concerns begin to arise. However, it's important for you to realize that the panic you feel at first is a normal part of the adaptation process—and it will pass.

Analysis Paralysis

Closely related to panic is "analysis paralysis." People who are more analytically inclined sometimes find that they get so involved in trying to figure out the "whys," "hows," and "what-ifs" that they can think of little else. The problem with this condition is that it's impossible to move forward, and to be a positive role model for your children, friends, and family.

Anger

Unfortunately, these initial reactions will most likely give way to other "normal" but unpleasant emotions. There's a blurry line between the initial panic and subsequent anger, but most parents experience anger early on. It's not directed at your child, of course, and it's completely normal. Some people are angry at God or Fate. This may be especially true for parents whose child has additional (sometimes accompanying) conditions such as Down syndrome or diabetes and can't understand what their child did to deserve this double helping of medical problems. Some parents are angry at the pediatricians who sent them away telling them their child was fine. Many are angry at food manufacturers who feel compelled to add malt flavoring to every cereal they make, and who won't just make it simple by putting "gluten" on the ingredients list. Some are even angry at whomever passed the "defective gene" to their child.

It's important to recognize your anger as a normal part of adaptation, but also to develop appropriate outlets for it. Some people benefit from having someone to talk to; others feel better if they can write in a journal or have another type of artistic outlet. Still others simply throw themselves actively into the task at hand. Whatever your coping style, be sure to put some effort into taking care of yourself. You will need to be the guiding force for the changes in your child's life.

Remember that your child will likely be angry, too, even if he's too young to understand the diagnosis. He may be angry at you for taking away the foods he enjoys, or angry that he feels deprived. Older children often feel anger at the same people and circumstances that adults experience: anger at the relative who passed on the gene; anger at God; anger at food manufacturers.

Help your child deal with anger in an appropriate manner. Let him talk, draw angry pictures, or do whatever else helps him feel as though he's being heard. Listen carefully. Tell him you understand, and that he has every right to feel angry. But make sure he understands that you are there to help him, and that together you will learn how to live a happy, healthy gluten-free life.

Some kids feel no anger whatsoever. This too is normal, and should not be considered to be apathy, repression, or any other "abnormal" response.

Grief

Most parents do experience grief with regard to their child's diagnosis. As mentioned above, grief is a very normal response to any perceived loss. You may feel sad at the thought that your child's life won't be absolutely perfect, or because you worry that he may be teased or may experience health problems.

"Deanna was diagnosed six years ago. At first I felt so sad—sad for her, sad for myself, and sad for the rest of the family. As I learned to handle the diet, I felt better about things. But every couple of years, as she goes through different phases of her life and her diet causes various challenges for her, I find myself feeling sad again. I wonder if it is normal to feel this way, especially so long after the original diagnosis."

—Sarah M.

It is very important to recognize your grief and to allow yourself a grieving period. Difficult emotions tend to become more manageable when dealt with directly than when they are ignored. However, it is also important not to dwell on it. Your own attitude about your child's health will have a significant impact on his attitude about himself. Grief is one of the emotions that may rear its ugly head every couple of years and must be addressed again each time.

Denial

Denial is a common emotion that may occur a few months after your child has been on a gluten-free diet and is doing better. Nearly everyone says that their child starts looking so good, feeling so healthy, that they start to suspect that maybe there was never anything wrong in the first place! Sometimes parents whose kids are suspected of having celiac disease will be told to "challenge" their kids and put them back on gluten. They sometimes find that when they do this, their child doesn't appear to show any response to gluten. This is typical, and so is your probable (but overly hopeful and erroneous) conclusion that your child doesn't actually have celiac disease.

Denial often occurs again when your child is older—ten years old or so. Usually the reason it occurs at this stage is because your child may get some gluten, whether accidentally or because he cheated, and will have no response (see information on the "Honeymoon Period," page163. It is common for parents and kids both to eagerly assume the child has "outgrown" the condition, or that he never had it, and was misdiagnosed. Be cautious about jumping to conclusions. Chances are, the diagnosis was correct, and, no, children *don't* grow out of it.

The danger in this stage is that there's the temptation to cheat—to go ahead and give the child gluten, since he "probably doesn't have any 'conditions' anyway!" Don't do it. This denial phase too will pass, and reality will set in.

Fear and Heartache

Fear and heartache seem to go hand in hand. Every time your child has a tummy ache (and all kids get them, remember), you'll wonder if he's gotten some gluten. You may even be afraid that you aren't following the diet closely enough. Try not to become consumed with fear. Deal with it together as a family; this will help you relax.

The anguish you feel on your kid's behalf may raise questions that can haunt you: Will this make him less appealing as a husband? Will he be traumatized and psychologically impaired? Will his friends make fun of him? Can I handle the sorrow if they do? Can he? If he has autism or another diagnosis such as Down syndrome or diabetes, will his condition affect his ability to live independently as an adult? What will his future bring? Relax. These thoughts disappear as you *and* your child become more comfortable with the diet and realize that a "normal life" is made up of much more than food.

Self-Pity

Another normal-but-unpleasant emotion you may experience is self-pity. Here you have a child who has been sick, who has a condition he will never outgrow, and you're feeling sorry for yourself. Don't feel guilty about that!

Nearly every parent feels some self-pity shortly after embarking upon the GF lifestyle. And why not? All the other parents get to whip up a quick box of macaroni-and-cheese for dinner, drive through a fast food restaurant without making several calls beforehand, and shove a bunch of crackers in the kid's fist when he's whining in the car. *Their* biggest dietary concern is making sure their kids' pizza has enough pepperoni on it to count as a source of protein. So go ahead—feel a little sorry for yourself, because it *is* tough. But then get over it and move on, because your family needs you. Besides, you have some work to do to prepare yourself—and your child—for a happy, healthy gluten-free life.

Guilt

Many parents are guilt-ridden, and will ask, "What did I do to give my child this condition?" Beyond the basic physiology of the birds and the bees, the answer is *nothing*. Certainly you did nothing *wrong*. Celiac disease and many of the other conditions discussed in this book are genetic conditions, so there *is* a biological connection, and in those cases, someone *did* pass a gene along to the child. But there is certainly no reason to wallow in guilt, because nothing could have been done differently to avoid the condition.

Acceptance

Yes, you will learn to accept the diagnosis, and you will one day look back and wonder why it seemed so overwhelming at first. While some of the other emotions may rear their ugly heads again from time to time, you will realize that it's a lot more fun to focus on your child's activities, school projects, friends, sports, accomplishments, and virtues than it is to spend your energy worrying about a "label" he was given.

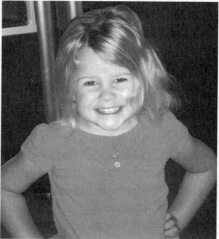

Am I Doing Something Wrong? It Seems Too Easy . . .

Ah, this is when you know you've finally made it.

There comes a time when parents who have become accustomed to dealing with their child's gluten-free diet wonder if they're doing something wrong because it seems too easy. Those feelings of self-doubt are usually triggered by a conversation with a parent who is still in the panic phase—still trying to figure out what, besides Fritos, they can feed their child, and how their lives will ever return to "normal." The experienced parent will think, "Gee, I really don't give any thought to it anymore. I wonder if I'm being too lax, or if I'm missing something here. It's just really not that tough."

When this happens to you, don't question yourself. Just enjoy the peace of mind, and realize you have acclimated to your new lifestyle. With the realization that you have that monkey off your back, you may want to take some time to help someone else with a difficult situation, and revel in the satisfaction that will bring.

6

Attitude Is Life... Deal with It; Don't Dwell on It

> "Annie was just diagnosed last week, and I find myself coddling her, trying to make up for the diagnosis in some way. I'm still reeling with emotion, and I feel overwhelmed. Will it ever get easier?"
>
> —Darryl S.

Feeding the kiddos is crucial (how's that for overstating the obvious?!), and this book is designed to give you all the tools and information you need to make sure you find plenty of delicious, nutritious options that are safe for your child to eat.

But beyond the food is the mood. Yours. And it's really important, because for most of you, this is a for-the-rest-of-your-child's-life deal. The last chapter talked about some emotions you're likely to feel or have felt. This chapter sheds some light on how you can get beyond some of the stumbling blocks you might be encountering.

Keep It In Perspective

Deal with it; don't dwell on it: That's my mantra throughout this book. I've seen many parents over the years get so caught up with the "inconveniences" of having a gluten-free child that it becomes a negative, controlling force in their lives. Yes, it's difficult at first, and it *is* a family affair, affecting everyone in the family greatly. But how you deal with it is going to influence your child's

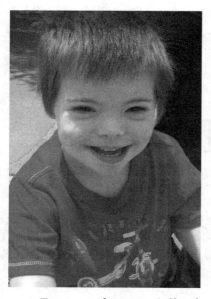

emotions and behavior, and can have long-lasting effects. Remember, your child's diet is a small part of her life; it shouldn't be the entire focus.

Shortly after diagnosis of celiac disease, children are usually experiencing many physical and emotional changes. Chances are, if your child has celiac disease, she was very sick or had difficult behavioral challenges. You were probably doting over her, in some cases genuinely concerned about whether she was even going to live through the ordeal. That has probably created some interesting dynamics: you had a sick child, and in some cases, it was grave; it will be difficult for you to let go of that fear and concern at first. As for your child, she has been getting a lot of attention from parents and doctors, and may have mixed emotions about getting better!

Fortunately, especially if your child has celiac disease or gluten sensitivity, you should see fairly quick improvement in her physical health once you start a gluten-free diet. And although most physicians agree that there are behavioral issues when a child with celiac disease is still on a gluten-containing diet, many of these, if not all, will disappear quickly after beginning a gluten-free diet.

There will, however, be periods of frustration and irritability, and the temptation to let her have a birthday cupcake or holiday cookie. This may be especially true for those of you with kids with autism or Down syndrome, since they tend to have a difficult time giving up their favorite goodies! Hang in there, and whatever you do, don't let her cheat! Not only will it cause physical harm, but it is sending her a signal that you are going to be inconsistent about enforcing her diet. The entire family needs to take this diet very seriously, and you must commit yourselves to being 100 percent gluten-free.

Be supportive during these periods of frustration; let your child know her feelings are completely normal. But urge her, especially by example, to move forward, discovering the wonderful new world of gluten-free living.

Be Optimistic, Even If You Have to Fake It at First

Have you ever pretended to feel a certain way, for whatever reason, and found that eventually you *actually feel* that way? It's a wonderful power that our brains have, and most of us are not even aware of it. Of course, it can be used for positive feelings or negative ones, but for the purpose of this book, we'll focus on "pretending" to be optimistic.

Try thinking of the diagnosis and your child's condition as a challenge. Don't let it knock you down (at least not for long). Come up with reasons to think of this as a good thing—maybe it's bringing you and your child, or you and your spouse, closer together. Maybe it's causing you to focus on a healthier diet. Perhaps it's forcing you to focus less on work and more on your family. If you need to, write down the reasons that this could be a good thing in your life. Memorize them. Believe them. You will be amazed at how your behavior and sincere feelings will follow.

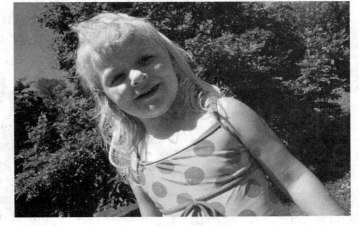

The truth is that the diagnosis of celiac disease in our children is far harder on us parents than it is on our children. We tend to think of the things *we* ate as children. We tend to focus on what they're *missing*. But you know what? They don't *know* what they're missing! You could be feeding them daffodils every day, and they wouldn't know what they were missing out on. Sure, at first they know, especially if they're older. But after they adjust to their lifestyle, it's nothing more than a "cultural" difference. Vegetarians don't eat meat. They don't focus on the steak and pork chops they're missing; they take pleasure in the wonderful assortment of foods that they do enjoy.

It's our disappointment for our children that makes this so difficult—so learn to see the positive, and it will be reflected in your child's optimistic views and behaviors. Remember that a positive attitude for life begins in their earliest years.

They **Are** Different, and That's Okay!

When parents of kids new to the diet contact me, one of the first things they always say is, "I'm so worried she'll grow up feeling *different* from the other kids."

It's a natural response. As adults, we have all felt "different" at one time or another, and that feeling has made us feel uncomfortable. We make the assumption that feeling "different" is painful. As parents, we want to spare our children the heartache that we *anticipate* they'll feel.

The fact is, they *are* different—but no different from someone with an allergy to chocolate or peanuts. No different from the child whose recess activities are limited due to asthma. No different from the child with a different religious or ethnic background.

> *"I'm afraid people will treat Jenna differently because her diet may seem strange to them. I don't want her to feel abnormal. What can I do to make it so she doesn't feel so different?"*
>
> —Mike J.

Our children need to know that they *are* different, and that's okay. If you lead them to believe they're *no* different from anyone else, they're surely going to wonder why *everyone else* eats such peculiar stuff. It will skew their entire sense of reality, because the reality is that *they* are the ones with the "different" diet. They need to learn to deal with that. It's not a bad thing, nor is it anything to shield them from.

Don't Keep Her in a Bubble

> *"It seems like we can't even venture out of the house. We're afraid to go out to dinner, to send him to school, or to let him go to friends' houses. Will we ever be able to get out of the house?!"*
>
> —Scott W.

It's natural to want to protect your child, and it may take some time to feel comfortable enough with the diet to venture out. It may seem at first that you need to forego dinner at friends' houses or restaurants. You may think you should eliminate travel from your activities, keep your child home while the other kids go away to camp, or tell her she can't go to a pizza party.

Don't do that to yourself or to your kids. Yes, every time you venture outside the safety of your gluten-friendly kitchen, you're taking a risk that she will get some gluten. And yes, it's important to be as diligent as you can about ensuring a 100 percent gluten-free diet. So how do you resolve that paradox? You could keep your child in a bubble—but I think it's worse to grow up in isolation than to take the risk that she may get a small bit of gluten. It's important to remember an almost universal goal of raising children: to teach our kids to live successfully in the world. To learn about their world, they have to be immersed in it.

Teach Your Child to Have a Positive Attitude

Attitudes are contagious. So the first and most important thing is to remember that your child is *always* watching how you handle situations—and you can bet she'll be tuning in to how you deal with her condition.

Tell your child that *she is in control of how she feels*. She can choose to feel sad, or she can choose to feel happy. Of course, we all feel sad sometimes, and sadness is perfectly justified when you're first finding out you have dietary restrictions. It's important that your child understands that, and isn't *too* quick to shrug off

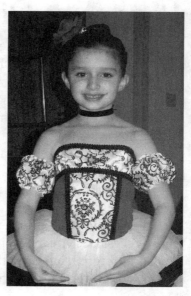

or bury negative emotions. Some of the most important lessons children learn involve managing emotions, especially "unpleasant" ones.

Your child may feel sad when she can't eat something the other kids are eating, or when a friend or relative "just doesn't get it." Sympathize, but don't let her dwell on it. Teach her that she can *choose* to pull herself out of that gloomy feeling by thinking of how lucky she is to be able to eat chocolate or other yummy things that some people can't eat. Help her focus on the positive things—not only concerning her diet, but positive attributes that she has or exciting things going on in her life.

Being on a gluten-free diet isn't that bad—in fact, I actually don't mind it! Having Celiac disease can be hard sometimes, I'll most certainly admit, but it also has many bonuses! The kids at school are always stuck eating the same old cafeteria food, but I can have anything from lasagna to crab cakes to steak or salad! The guys (A.K.A. my friends) are always begging me for a part of my lunch because it A) looks SOOO good OR B) Smells SOOO good!

Holidays can be hard, though. I'm always wishing that I could have all the different types of candy on Halloween, instead of the select few. But hey, SOME candy is better then NO candy, am I right? And you would be surprised on how many different kinds of candy is O.K.! Baby Ruth's, Almond Joys, Three Musketeers, and Reese's Peanut Butter Cups, just to name a very few!

On another matter, kids with celiac live pretty normal lives. I can hang out with my friends, build tree forts, play XBox, and go to the store and get some soda pop (I just have to be careful what kind). In other words, we are not handicapped, and we are not weak because of our restricted diet. We are regular people!

—Wyatt M., age 12

Don't Make a Big Deal of It to Her

Other than discussing food choices and other practical matters associated with the gluten-free lifestyle, try not to make this a huge issue in your life. Of course it *is*, but for your child's sake, pretend it isn't. Sometimes it's tough not to make a big deal of it, because you assume that it will have the same impact on your child's life as it has on yours. It doesn't. For the most part, sports or activities, school, and friends are what kids want to think about—and what they *should* be thinking about.

A couple of times, in an attempt to be sensitive and communicative, we have tried asking Tyler how it makes him feel to have celiac disease. We expected to hear how emotionally devastating it is, how angry he is at that unknown descendant who passed him the "inferior" gene. Instead, he looked at us as though we had the I.Q. of an oyster, and said, "It doesn't feel like anything. It's no big deal."

Don't Let Her Feel Like a Burden— Obvious? Not Always

"Don't let your child feel like a burden" sounds like elementary psychology, and appears to be blatantly obvious. But picture yourself at the end of a long week, tired from a busy day, ready to relax, and you hear, "Mommy, I don't have any bread left. Can we make some?" Surely you'll be tempted to roll your eyes and sigh—a perfectly natural reaction, but not as subtle as you may think, and likely not to be overlooked by your child. This is where you'll be cursing all of your friends who can just make a quick trip to the grocery store. Go ahead and curse them, but do it to yourself.

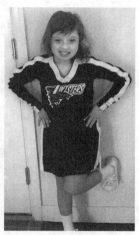

The last thing you want is for your child to think that she is causing you extra stress because of her diet. Kids are so perceptive! You don't have to say anything. They'll read it in your eyes, or your body language, especially if they're looking for it because they've suspected in the past that their diet creates a burden. Muster any energy you have left, give her a big smile, and pull out the trusty bread maker. (Or offer a yummy alternative.)

Celiac Disease Is Not a Four-Letter Word

I realize a lot of you have kids who don't have celiac disease, but are gluten-free for other reasons. This section pertains to you, too—but I've written it to address the specific diagnosis of celiac disease because it's such a common and perplexing frustration we share.

> *"Christopher had chronic diarrhea, and because celiac disease runs in our family, we suggested to our pediatrician that he should do an antibody screening. But he said that because Christopher was normal height and weight, there was no reason to test him. Why won't he just do the test?"*
>
> —Lynnette C.

Although celiac disease is not a four-letter word, people sure do *act* like it is! What is it about this condition that makes people squirm? Relatives can have every classic symptom, yet they refuse to be tested. It can't be that the condition involves the "insides," and is therefore too private in nature. After all, people are happy to discuss their Crohn's disease, ulcerative colitis, hair loss, prostate problems, and infertility. No, it's something much less tangible and much more subtle.

> *"Some people would rather hear that they have to take a pill every day of their lives, than to hear that they have to change their diet!"*
> —Elaine Monarch, Celiac Disease Foundation

Even many doctors are hesitant to accept celiac disease. I have seen several cases in which celiac disease runs in the family, and a child has classic symptoms; parents ask for their child to be tested, and the doctor refuses. WHY? The blood test is not expensive, it's noninvasive, and it's an excellent initial screening. But there's something about celiac disease that people want to avoid.

Be aware of this fact, but don't buy into it. There is nothing to be ashamed of, and nothing to be embarrassed about. While there is no need to wear a badge of celiac disease, be aware of how your child may be picking up on the stigma, and be careful that your child never feels as though her condition is something to hide.

Realize You Have New Commitments

Your new gluten-free (and maybe casein-free) lifestyle will require you to spend more time preparing, planning, cooking, educating, and volunteering your time.

The best way to help your child ease into a gluten-free lifestyle is for you to volunteer as often as you can to help with, if not lead, school-related and extracurricular activities. If you can, chaperone field trips and camping expeditions or volunteer to help with lunch time at school. (But do this only if your school has volunteers; you don't want to be the one parent there—it may make your child feel even more "different.")

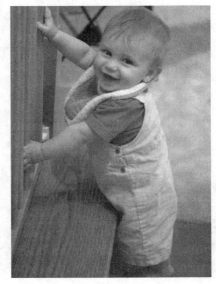

Divide this extra effort between husband and wife, if possible. Dads are just as good (or better) at chaperoning on field trips as moms are! It's your job to do everything in your power to keep your child happy and healthy. When you have a child with dietary restrictions, that may mean putting in a little extra effort at times.

7

Should the Entire Family Be Gluten-Free?

"I don't want David to see the rest of the family eating things that he can't eat, so I'm thinking about getting rid of everything in the house that has gluten in it, and making the entire house gluten-free. Would that make it easier for him to deal with the diet?"

—Cindy P.

Nearly every family that has a member who is on a strict, gluten-free diet considers turning the entire house into a gluten-free zone. Is it necessary to do so? Is it "easier" on everyone? Well, it is definitely not *necessary* for the entire family to be gluten-free. There are, in fact, pros and cons to both sides.

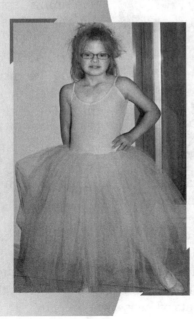

The Pros

The pros of having an entirely gluten-free family are that it's simpler at menu-planning time, shopping is less cumbersome, it's easier to keep a gluten-free kitchen, there is little or no possibility of accidental contamination or ingestion, and there's no temptation for your child to cheat (at home). You also avoid the resentment that your gluten-free child may feel when the rest of the family is eating something that he can't eat.

The Cons

Remember, in solving one problem, you can create another. If the entire family goes gluten-free, your nongluten-free kids (and spouse!) may begin to resent the gluten-free child for imposing the diet on the family.

Perhaps the most resounding argument against having the entire family lead a completely gluten-free lifestyle is that *it simply isn't reality*. Kids who are gluten-free (especially those who *have* to be gluten-free for life because of celiac disease) have to learn to live in a gluten-laden world. Yes, menu-planning is more difficult when you have to cook "both ways," and yes, the child on the gluten-free diet is likely to feel pangs of jealousy and even isolation. But there are ways to soften those blows, yet still live in a "real" world surrounded by gluten. What better place to teach your child those important life's lessons than in the safe, loving, controlled environment of your own home?

Finding a Happy Medium

Perhaps the best compromise is to have the family be *relatively* gluten-free. Try to eat the same types of meals, with a small portion being different when necessary.

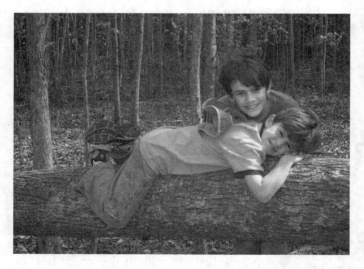

For instance, if it's spaghetti night, you might want to make gluten-free pasta for everyone. But if not, it's okay to have everyone eat gluten-containing spaghetti with the one child eating gluten-free pasta (be sure to use separate pots, colanders, and serving utensils—see the cooking chapter for more on that). The entire family can use the same GF spaghetti sauce and toppings, and people will hardly notice that one child is eating a different type of pasta. Just make sure that your child's meal and the family's meal are pretty much the same. You don't want to be eating lasagna and offering him lima beans.

Try to find GF staple items that everyone likes—yogurt, salad dressings, condiments, sauces, and other frequently used foods and accompaniments. That way the possibility of cross-contamination or accidental gluten ingestion is minimized, your gluten-free child doesn't feel ostracized, and you won't need to convert the spare bedroom into a pantry to accommodate two sets of every type of food.

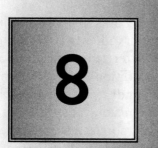

8

Talking to Your Child about Her Condition

"Tiffany was diagnosed a month ago. She's only three years old, and I figured she was too young to understand, so I've just been taking charge of her diet and I haven't talked to her about gluten sensitivity. I thought maybe I'd wait until she's five or six. My husband thinks we should do it now. What's the right age?"
—Lynn and John T.

In most cases, talking to your kids about their diet should start from Day One. After all, much of their life involves putting food into their mouths—it's important that the food is safe. Just as you'd teach them any safety rule at the earliest age possible, you should discuss their diet as early as possible, as well. But when you discuss their medical conditions depends upon what their conditions are and how apt they are to grasp the concepts.

Educating Your Child

Whether your child is two or twelve, you need to start talking to her about her diet *now*. Don't use made-up words, and don't be afraid to use big words. Understanding is a tool that benefits both children and adults, although the extent of information provided will vary with the age of your child. It's important to *give your child both an understanding and control of her diet so the diet doesn't control her!*

Regardless of her age and depending upon her condition, your child is most likely aware that she has been sick, gone through testing, her parents have been concerned, and that doctors have been doing all sorts of crazy things to her. Once the diagnosis is established, it's time to explain to her that all of that is behind her now, and that she's going to start feeling a lot better, starting right away!

Open the conversation by explaining that she has a condition that requires a gluten-free diet. How extensive this conversation will be depends upon the age of your child, of course, but give her as much information as she seems to want.

Don't pout, cry, or look sad or apologetic when you talk about it! Explain matter-of-factly that some people can't eat sugar, others can't eat chocolate, and she can't eat gluten. Surely you know someone who has a dietary restriction that you can point out as an example. Keep remembering, and expressing to her, that the *good* thing is she's going to start feeling better right away!

When you first start talking about gluten, make sure you have a quick "sound bite" to describe it. For instance, you might say, "You can't eat gluten. Gluten is in wheat, oats, rye, and barley." (You might want to add "malt" to the list, too. Malt is made from barley, but how many kids *or* adults know that?) Every time you refer to "gluten," try to follow it up with the identical phrase: "gluten is in wheat, oats, rye, and barley (malt)." Repeat the phrase every time the key word (gluten) is mentioned, and, even if your child doesn't have a clue what these things are, she'll learn the words. This is useful so that she will be able to repeat them to others as necessary. It's important that she can say the words, even if she doesn't understand what they mean.

If Your Child Has a Disability

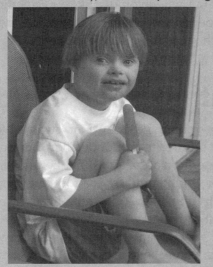

If your child has difficulty communicating due to Down syndrome, autism, or another disability, consider providing her with a card that explains that she can't eat wheat, oats, rye, and barley (malt). Over time, teach her to show it to people who may offer her food. For example, when your child goes to a friend's house, have her offer the card to the parent in charge.

In the beginning, you may need to use hand-over-hand guidance to prompt her to show the card at appropriate times. As time goes on, you might prompt her with the word "card" or wait to see whether she will remember to show the card on her own. The goal is for her to eventually be independent in recognizing people who need to know about the foods she cannot eat.

If your child uses an alternative or augmentative communication system, include information about your child's food restrictions in her communication system. That way, she can just press the button or icon on her communication device to explain what she can or can't eat, or turn to the appropriate page in her communication book.

It is through actions such as telling others about the disease that your child will begin managing her own condition. Of course, it is also important to talk with your child about what items *contain* gluten, such as cookies, bread, and cereal. But getting her to think and talk in "sound bites" or offer an explanatory card (see sidebar) will help her communicate her condition and restrictions to others, even before she fully understands the complexities of the diet.

How You Might Bring It Up with Your Young Child

It's a lot easier to explain medical conditions such as celiac disease to older children than to younger ones (although older kids pose additional challenges in terms of cheating), so we have outlined an example of how you might begin to explain the condition and gluten to younger kids. To simplify, we've focused these pretend conversations on celiac disease. If your child has a different condition, you'll need to edit the conversations a tad. Remember, keep that positive attitude!

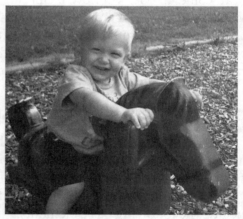

Ages 1-6: "Honey, you know we've been going to see Dr. B. a whole bunch lately, right? Well, he is *so* smart that he figured out what we can do to make you feel better!" (Keep that smile and enthusiasm!) "See, you have this thing called celiac disease. That's why you weren't feeling good, but now that we know what it is, you're going to start feeling much better! Celiac disease just means there are some things you can't eat, but there are *lots* of things you *can* eat! Let's go in the pantry right now and find some gluten-free snacks together."

At this point, let her point out something she wants. Chances are, she'll pick something with gluten. Now's your chance to say, "Oh, that looks really yummy. But that has gluten in it—gluten is in wheat, oats, rye, and barley (malt). Let's see what we have that doesn't have gluten in it. . . ." (This is when you pick up a gluten-free candy bar or something *really* yummy that you've stashed for this very moment.)

Of course, your discussions will evolve, and there is a steep learning curve for everyone involved. Many of the implications of having a dietary restriction do not become immediately clear. Many such issues will emerge gradually over time and will require learning and adaptation for some time to come. For instance, you just learned something new—Rule Number One—from the monologue above: always have an alternative (and better tasting) snack handy. But we'll talk more about that in later chapters.

Teach with Familiar Examples

When you're trying to explain to your child that gluten is in wheat, oats, rye, and barley (malt), remember that she probably doesn't know exactly what those words mean. One technique to help her understand the meaning of the words is to link each grain with a product she knows. For instance, "Wheat is in the bread we used to eat. It's also in crackers, spaghetti, cakes, and cookies. But now we'll be eating special cookies (bread, spaghetti, etc.) that don't have any wheat in them."

Activities for Young Kids

Activities are an effective learning tool for young children, and a great way for young kids to become involved in the process of learning about the gluten-free diet. It's a good idea to involve all of your children in the activities, even those who are not on a GF diet. Not only will they learn about the diet too, but it will help all family members feel that "we're all in this together."

There are activity books available that are geared toward the gluten-free child, or you can come up with your own. One suggestion is to have your child help you make a food booklet or flashcards with "good" foods and "bad" foods. Cooking magazines and old cookbooks are loaded with colorful pictures. You can paste the pictures onto colored paper or colorful cloth scraps, and bind them together with yarn or rings that snap closed. You can even use the booklet as a resource for friends and family!

"Just the Facts, Ma'am" Approach for Older Kids

How you talk with your older child depends upon the relationship you have and the responses you get throughout the conversation. Basically, though, older kids would prefer you just cut to the chase.

Your child is going to want the basic facts. Elaborate as you'd like, but remember to include the following basic elements:

- ◆ You have celiac disease.
- ◆ This is what celiac disease is.
- ◆ That's why you haven't felt well.
- ◆ People with celiac disease can't eat gluten.
- ◆ Gluten is in wheat, oats, rye, and barley (malt).
- ◆ Here are some lists of things that are okay to eat, and things that are not.
- ◆ If you get even a tiny bit of gluten, it does really bad things to you internally.
- ◆ You need to learn how to say, "No thank you."
- ◆ If you don't know for sure, don't eat it.
- ◆ It may not be easy, but we'll help you through it.

Your discussions with older kids are important, but it's even more important to help them research the condition on their own. The more they know, the less scary it will be, and learning about it is the first step in taking responsibility for their own health. Many older children question anything their parents tell them until it is verified by another source. There are a number of good websites and various written materials that can help.

It is important for you to understand that, shortly after being diagnosed, older children may go through many of the same emotions that parents experience (described in Chapter Five). If you're aware of these normal-but-not-always-pleasant emotions, you will likely be more patient and supportive during your interactions with your child.

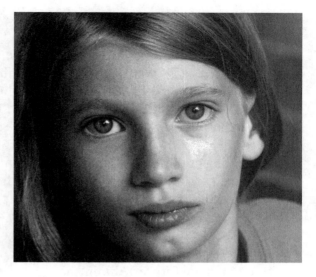

"If You Feel Bad, You Must Have Gotten Gluten"

Talking with your child about her condition is an ongoing process—something you discuss in different ways as her level of understanding (and yours) grows. I do *not* want to give the impression that you should dwell on the subject, nor should you make a huge deal out of it (in fact, I believe quite the opposite). But there are some things you want to "condition in," so to speak.

For instance, especially in the beginning, when you refer to gluten, you need to remind your child that she can't eat gluten. You might want to say something like, "Remember, you can't eat gluten. It makes you feel icky." (Okay, if she's thirteen, you may want to choose a word other than "icky.") You may feel like you're being redundant, repetitive, and even a nag. And you *are!* But think about how many dozens of times you've said, "Don't run with a sucker in your mouth," and yet 99 percent of the time when your kids put a sucker in their mouth, it's as though their transmission automatically kicks into "RUN" mode. Some things are so important that they just have to be repeated. It may not be that your child forgot, or even that she's intentionally defying or ignoring you—it's that her knowledge of that association hasn't gone to a deep, subliminal level yet.

It may be helpful to think about how associations between events are developed. Some associations are conditioned in very early. For instance, cry = attention from a parent. Mommy talking on phone = ask for something and chances are good that you'll get it. These aren't associations that children are consciously aware of. Rather, these associations develop through observation. In other words, they are conditioned by experience. Children observe that, sure enough, when Mommy has that phone on her ear and is deep in conversation, she tends to nod when interrupted and asked a question. The same type of process is necessary for conditioning your child that "gluten makes you feel icky." You want this lesson to be so ingrained in her head that she comes to believe it, deep down inside, at the level where her subconscious is also supposed to be chanting, "hit brother = time-out."

The key words in the last sentence were, "comes to believe it." If your child is younger than a teen, you still have some influence over what she believes. This is where conditioning comes in again. I believe there is great power in conditioning your child to believe that gluten makes her feel icky. The truth is, eating gluten is not *always* going to make her feel icky, and this can create some difficulties when you're trying to convince her how awful gluten is for her body. So, in an effort to maximize your child's understanding of this unpleasant reality, you may want to take advantage of any time she *does* feel icky, and blame it on gluten. With this necessary goal in mind, it doesn't really matter if it's the flu, a "regular ol' tummy ache," food poisoning, or a mild headache. When she complains of symptoms, reply with, "Oh, honey, I am so sorry to hear you don't feel well. Maybe you accidentally got some gluten. It makes you feel icky, you know." As the association becomes clearer, the likelihood that she will try to sneak some gluten in the future is diminished.

Read Labels Together—Even If She Can't Read Yet

Whether your child can read or not, it is important to read the product labels together. I know that sounds silly. If she can't read, why would you have her read a label with you? The answer is dual purpose. Reading labels with your child not only involves her in the decision-making process, it also helps her get in the habit of looking at labels on packages. It's that conditioning thing again.

Of course, you don't ask her to read the words aloud to you, but you can hold the package together, point to each word on the ingredients list, and when you get to, for instance, "wheat," you say, "wheat—nope. Can't eat wheat, because wheat has gluten in it." You may even want to finish with, "Gluten makes you feel icky." Your continual and repetitive statements of these basic concepts really will help increase your child's understanding of, and belief in, the impact of gluten on her body. Repetition is a fundamental aspect of the conditioning process.

I knew I had celiac disease when I was 18 months old. Sometimes you can feel mad because you want other people's food. If somebody ever offers you some food say "No thank you." Try your best and do not eat any rye, malt, barley, or wheat. I love being a celiac because it is super fun!

—Megan R., age 7

How to Say "No Thank You"

Unfortunately, there *will* be the well-meaning friend or relative who slips your child a cookie and says with a conspiratorial wink, "Don't tell Mommy and Daddy." There will also be people who are completely unaware of your child's condition, and, with the best of intentions, will offer her something she can't eat. At holidays, it seems as if people come swarming from nowhere to offer children candy canes or other treats that may or may not be safe.

It is very important to talk with your child about temptation and why people will tempt her. Explain that Grandpa means well, but that he just doesn't understand how bad gluten is for her. Tell her that the elves offering cookies at the mall just don't know that she can't eat those things. But remind her of how very important it is not to eat things that might have gluten in them.

Teach her to say, "No thank you" without apology, explanation, or embarrassment. There are times when saying anything further can be awkward and it certainly isn't necessary. Of course if she *wants* to explain, that's fine. But stress that it's okay to politely refuse the treat. And if you're there, be sure to offer a tasty alternative.

Let Her Know There Are Alternatives: Do the "Treat Trade"

When discussing your child's dietary restrictions, make sure she knows that there are always tasty alternatives. Be sure to reinforce this with your actions. You may have to get creative sometimes, and short notice can be a real curse—but it's important to always offer some sort of an alternative when your child is in a situation in which she

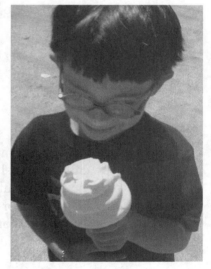

can't eat something. For instance, if the other kids are eating birthday cupcakes and you didn't have time to make gluten-free cupcakes, offer her a candy bar. If the other kids are eating Christmas cookies, make sure she has her favorite treat available. When you see the disappointment on her face because all the other kids get to have pizza, make her her favorite meal—preferably her gluten-free pizza. This technique is most effective if the alternative is similar to what the other kids are eating.

It can also help if the alternative is just a little bit "better" than what the other kids get. When the other kids in Tyler's class were eating birthday cake and he got a candy bar, they all complained that he always got the "good" stuff!

How the food looks is just as important as how it tastes. If the other kids are having a pizza party and you send your child with her own pizza, it better look "right." If not, you can be sure she will hide it, toss it, and come home famished and embarrassed.

Okay, It's Time to Eat!

So you've had your little heart-to-heart, and your child is saying, "Yeah, yeah, whatever. Celiac schmeliac. Let's EAT!" Start by asking her to choose a food she'd like to eat. After she chooses something, ask her if she thinks it has gluten in it. Remind her that gluten is in wheat, oats, rye, and barley (malt). Yes, of course I know that she doesn't know what these things are! That's not the point! The point is that in asking her this question you are encouraging her to think about what she can and can't eat.

Let her choose a few items, and if they contain gluten, point out why they're not okay to eat: "No, those cookies have flour in them. That means they have gluten." Give her a couple of tries, and then let her off the hook by "finding" something you've hidden away—the yummiest gluten-free treat you can think of! In the beginning, this activity should be at least a daily exercise, if not something you do every time she wants a snack. Repetition and familiarity are keys to getting started with this new lifestyle.

While the diagnosis is still fresh, she may be wondering if she's ever going to get a "normal" meal! It's important to explain that dinners *will* be a little different now, and be sure to involve her in the menu-planning process. This will be tough at first, at least until you've figured out how to prepare gluten-free pasta, pizza, and other highly requested menu items. But it is very important to her adaptation to at least let her *think* she's helping plan the menus, especially if there are things she happens to like that are gluten-free, such as salad or rice.

Most importantly, when you're teaching her about eating gluten-free, don't ever let her think that this dietary lifestyle is optional (if it's not for your child). Remind her that gluten will make her feel icky, and teach her the safest decision tool: "If you don't know, don't eat it."

Talking to the Other Kids in the Family

If there are siblings, it's important to talk with them about celiac disease and the new diet for the child with celiac disease. Depending upon the siblings' age(s) and relationships, they may have all sorts of questions, fears, and other feelings that need to be discussed. A diagnosis of one child in a family has an emotional impact on all family members. Be aware that your nondiagnosed children could be feeling any of the following emotions:

◆ Fear:
  ➤ Am I going to get it?
  ➤ Can I catch it?
  ➤ Is my brother/sister going to die?
◆ Resentment:
  ➤ She gets "special" attention and I don't.
  ➤ She gets better treats than I do (especially common when you're making a treat-trade and your child with celiac disease gets a really yummy treat).
  ➤ Parents care more about her than me because she's different.

"I know I need to talk to Renee's little brother about Renee's condition, but I'm afraid it might scare him. Will he be afraid she's going to die? Will he be afraid he has it too? How do we talk to the other kids in the family about this?"

—Rebecca B.

◆ Sadness or pity:
  ➤ She has a special diet and can't eat all of the really good stuff that many people can.

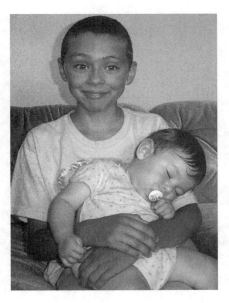

And then again, because siblings will be siblings, they may be tempted to make fun of her, tease her, or wave a greasy doughnut under her nose.

It's important for siblings to understand which foods are safe, which are not, and how important it is to take the diet seriously. Include them in all of your family discussions about your child's dietary needs, so that they too can make wise food choices for your child.

9

Give Your Child Control of His Diet!

"Jennifer just seems too young to be able to make the food choices that go along with the gluten-free diet. I feel more comfortable handling it myself. Besides, it's easier that way."

—Kristina T.

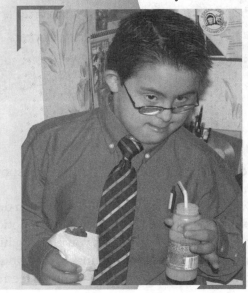

It's Your Responsibility to Give Your Child the Responsibility

It's funny. We teach our kids to dress themselves, to brush their own teeth, to go to the potty by themselves. . . . But when it comes to choosing what they eat, no sirree, Mommy will do that for you, thank you very much. Especially when the food they eat can make them very sick.

Yet, just as it's our job as parents to teach our children not to run out into the street, it's our responsibility to teach *them* to take responsibility for their diet. Remember, our job as parents, as difficult as it is for some of us to accept, is to raise our children in a loving, protective environment so that they can (ugh) *leave* us some day! Our instincts tell us to protect them, to control their environment so that nothing will hurt them. That's not too hard at three, but at thirteen, the very word "control" will drive a stake right through the heart of your relationship with your child.

It is important that children learn to size up risks and avoid or ignore them. They need to know that you trust them to take care of themselves—and you need to trust them to do so. However, getting to that point is a process that will take time for both sides.

As our children grow, they need to be able to:

◆ Identify, assess, and handle temptations and risks;
◆ Handle peer pressure;
◆ Handle social situations in which gluten is present;
◆ Prepare in advance for social functions in which there may be no gluten-free alternatives;
◆ Select foods in social settings and at the grocery store;
◆ Plan healthy, well-balanced gluten-free meals;
◆ Cook;
◆ Understand the consequences of cheating on the GF diet or accidental ingestion of gluten;
◆ Educate the people around them about celiac disease and the GF diet.

"Being gluten free is kind of a little sad at first, because you don't fit in. You don't eat the other kids' snacks. Like, say you're sitting next to your friend, who is not gluten free, and he offers you an extra chocolate chip cookie. You have to say no, because it's not gluten free. But then as you get more used to it, you get to have lots of fun. At parties, you have your own gluten-free cupcake (Mom makes the best cupcakes!). And people who are Boy Scouts can have most of the popcorn. And there's also gluten-free brownies, cookies, pizza, licorice, and they might even make gluten-free goldfish crackers—I think right now they're struggling to do that. I feel very good when I don't eat gluten.

—Micah W., age 8

It's Never Too Early

Whether your child is a toddler or a teen, let him know that he is responsible for his diet. *If he doesn't feel in control of his diet, his diet will control him.*

Of course your child's condition will dictate exactly how and when you do this, but helping your child to take control of his diet is crucial to his physical and emotional well-being, so you might as well start as soon as possible. Don't think you're doing him any favors by making all of his decisions for him, even if he is very young. In fact, you're taking away his sense of control, not to mention the fact that he's not learning to feed himself.

Remember the wise Native American saying: "If you give a person a fish, he will eat for a day. If you teach a person to fish, he will eat for a lifetime."

The earlier you give your child responsibility for his diet, the better off he'll be. It will also be easier for you in the long run. You will relax knowing that he understands the GF diet and can make responsible, healthy choices. More importantly, being responsible for his own diet will give your child confidence; he will know that he is capable of determining whether or not a food is gluten-free. In addition, at a subconscious level, he will have taken control of his condition, rather than letting it control him.

Things Children Can Do Right Away to Take Control

Menu Planning

Sometimes kids can be picky eaters—especially those experiencing food "jags," as kids on the autism spectrum often do. Toss into the equation the fact that your child's diet is severely limited, and meal planning can be frustrating, to say the least. Get your child involved in the meal-planning process! Not only will you be teaching him about the foods he can and can't eat, but you'll be working *together* to come up with a menu that pleases everyone. (The rule at our house is if you plan it, you eat it. No designating Tuesday as "fish night," and then deciding you don't like fish that week.) See Chapter 13 for menu suggestions.

Cooking

Kids are never too young to start helping in the kitchen. Of course, it's usually a lot easier and cleaner if they *don't* help, but it's important that children learn to prepare their own foods. Get all of the kids involved. A big part of the learning process, especially if you have other kids who are not gluten-free, is learning how to avoid contaminating utensils and cooking surfaces (see Chapter 11). By the time your child is eight, there will be many meals he can make on his own. The benefits are many: it makes it easier on you, it's fun for your children, and you're teach-

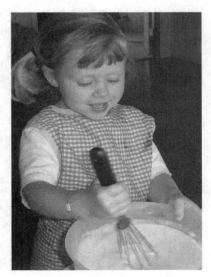

ing them to be independent. Remember, cleaning up the kitchen after you cook is one of the most important rules!

Packing Lunches

Have your child pack his own lunch, at least every now and then. You may want to check to make sure he doesn't go off to school with a solid meal of chips, candy bars, and "fruit" juice—but having him pack his own lunch will help you out and reinforce what he's learning about making good food choices. We offer gluten-free suggestions for lunches and other meals in Chapter 13.

Calling Manufacturers

Calling manufacturers to ask whether their products contain gluten is something that people on GF diets do frequently, so you might as well start involving your child at an early age. Fortunately, most large food manufacturers and distributors now have lists of gluten-free products, and can tell you over the phone whether or not their products are gluten-free. (A far cry from just a few years ago when even the most knowledgeable customer service reps would confidently respond to my inquiry about gluten, "Oh yes, honey, you may not know this, but gluten is another word for sugar. Most of our products *do* contain sugar and should be avoided by diabetics.")

Every now and then you'll get someone who hasn't heard of gluten, and you'll need to work your way to their quality control specialists, nutritionist, or dietitian. But for the most part, customer service reps who answer the phone can tell you whether or not their products contain gluten.

To help your child get the hang of this process, make sure his first few calls are to companies whose customer service reps have a gluten-free list in front of them. You'll want to scout out those companies in advance. Don't tell your child you've already called the company, because he'll feel you don't trust him and you'll deflate his sense of purpose. But when you've found a company with knowledgeable customer service reps at the other end, suggest to your child that he call about a product, and let him take it from there. Remind him to take notes and keep the information in a personalized product listing, as discussed in Chapter 12.

The Exceptions to the Rule

For some kids, it's just not practical to give them full or even partial control of their diet. Kids who have issues with self-control, or who don't have the cognitive skills to grasp the importance of strictly adhering to the diet still need to feel a sense of control, but not to the extent that I've described so far in this chapter.

You know your child best. Give him the credit for taking as much responsibility as he possibly can for the diet, and be sure to let him *feel* as though he's taking control.

Acknowledge the efforts he can make and is making, and empower him to continue and possibly even do more. The more power you give your child, the more responsible he feels—and acts.

Condition Your Child to Avoid Gluten

This entire chapter dealt with giving your child responsibility for his diet. But let go completely? No way! No matter how much "discussing," how much preaching, or how much begging you do, there's the possibility—read that as "likelihood"—that your child won't initially truly fathom the importance of always selecting safe, gluten-free foods. This almost always occurs in people with any type of dietary restriction.

Thanks to the wonders of the human body, you still have some tricks up your sleeve to help drive the point home, at least if your child experiences symptoms that are common with celiac disease or gluten sensitivity. There's often a simple built-in negative reinforcement clause—when he eats gluten, he feels bad.

Use this to your advantage! As I've mentioned earlier, I tricked my son when he was very young in an effort to condition him to avoid gluten. And it worked! Every time he hurt—whether it was a tummy ache, stubbed toe, or a headache, I said, "Uh oh, you must have gotten some gluten. We'll have to be more careful next time." In effect, I conditioned him to avoid gluten by teaching him that it caused discomfort. And for what it's worth, if the proof is in the gluten-free pudding: today I couldn't pay him to eat gluten.

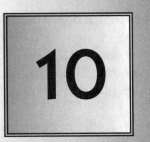

Dealing with Family and Friends

"I've tried to explain the GF diet to my family and friends, and they just don't seem to get it. Sometimes it seems like they're listening, and then they turn around and offer Kristy a piece of licorice that says 'wheat' right on the package. Am I doing something wrong?"
—Alex K.

You think it was tough talking to your kid about this diet and the reasons she's on it? Ha! Kids are quick studies compared to many adult relatives, friends, teachers, and other people you encounter.

Educating the adults in your life is, perhaps, one of the most difficult aspects of having a child on a gluten-free diet. Because there is so little awareness of celiac disease, autism, and other conditions that respond to a GF diet, responses from family and friends range from confusion (you'll recognize this response because as you're explaining it, their eyes glaze over and they say, "huh" a lot), to complete understanding (sorry, this is rare), to histrionic horror (usually exhibited by breaking down and sobbing at the word "disease"), to disbelief (particularly common if you're known to exaggerate from time to time).

Educate Your Family and Friends

You do not need to walk into a room and declare to everyone that your child is on a special diet. I say this facetiously, yet I've witnessed just that on more than a dozen occasions. Some parents feel that they're doing the right thing by letting everyone know about the dietary restriction, thereby reducing the chance that someone will slip their child a cookie. But keep in mind that your child is listening, and no matter how young she is, she can be embarrassed by such a declaration. Furthermore, many people just don't care or need to know.

Nevertheless, you *do* need to educate people who are in frequent contact with your child, or who may be in the position to give your child a meal or snack. Unfortunately, teaching others about the disease and gaining their true understanding isn't always easy. Other adults may go through a denial similar to what you experienced,

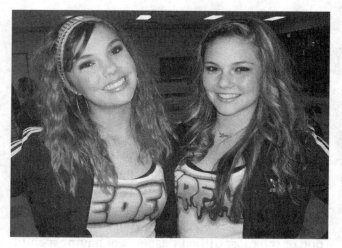

and, believe it or not, some people do not accept the existence of food allergies, sensitivities, or intolerances. And if your child is on the GF diet due to autism or related disorders, chances of people knowing about the possible relationship to gluten and casein is super slim. Given all this, prepare yourself, because mistakes *will* be made!

Be straightforward when you're talking with friends and family about your child's condition and diet, and keep your emotions in check. Your child will learn from you how *she* should educate others, so remember to be accurate, clear, and concise.

The easiest way to start educating your friends and family is to present them with a quick summary of what your child can and can't eat. You may want to give them a copy of this book and point out the chapters on allowed and forbidden ingredients or meal planning. Go over the information with the people you are talking to, and make sure they understand it thoroughly. Don't ignore the chapters that describe the medical conditions that may benefit from this diet. The more they understand, the more they're likely to accept and support.

As you're explaining it to them, carefully watch their responses, both verbal and nonverbal. It's important to recognize whether they're really "getting it" or not. If it appears that they do not fully understand the importance of this diet to your child's well-being, try rephrasing the information to help them out.

It's important to stress the severity of getting even a tiny bit of gluten—even if you have to get overly dramatic to make your point. If they're shrugging you off, or you get the impression they're taking it too lightly, use phrases such as, "Gluten is *toxic* to her system" or "Even a tiny bit can cause *lesions* internally." Nothing like the words "toxic" and "lesions" to make a point!

The Four Categories of Friends & Family

1. Those Who Handle It Well and "Get It"

You may be lucky enough to have a few friends or relatives who really "get it!" What a blessing. These people will really tune in when you break the news, they will ask lots of good questions, and will diligently study this book and any other information you give them. Some will even do some research on their own. When your child is planning to visit, they will stock up on gluten-free treats and will confidently plan gluten-free meals. These people are godsends to you—don't forget it, and more importantly, don't let them forget it!

"When I came over to my friend Jack's house for a sleepover, they were having pizza, so I brought my own little pizza, which was square. At dessert, we had root beer floats, and Jack's mom checked if it was gluten free just for me. And also in the morning, they had orange juice with pancakes. They checked if the orange juice was gluten free too. I brought my own pancakes that my Dad made. So I feel really good because people think about me."

—Micah W., age 8

2. Those Who Are Scared Even to Give Your Child a Piece of Fruit

"My best friend used to have Shari over all the time—our daughters are best friends. But now, she seems to be avoiding the opportunity to have her over, and I think it's because of Shari's diet. I'm a little angry about it, but I'm also wondering if there's something I should do?"

—Amy T.

It is important to realize that some of your friends will be afraid of harming your child! After all, you've told everyone how serious it can be for your child to get any gluten. Some of them may be scared to death to feed her. And they may not even be aware of their own fear, much less be able to communicate it tactfully to you.

Frankly, it's okay that they're afraid—better that than to have them be too nonchalant. It's up to you to be sensitive enough to understand how they're feeling, and to help them deal with their fear, even if they haven't said anything about it. Help them overcome their anxieties by providing menu ideas, suggesting fast food restaurants and appropriate food selections, and providing foods for your child when she is with that person. But be careful not to make it too easy on them, or they'll never learn.

3. Those Who Think You're Exaggerating

With some conditions, a "little" of the bad stuff is okay. It's okay, for instance, for diabetics to have a little sugar; it's okay for people on low-fat diets to have a little fat. So we need to understand that many people believe "a little is okay," and may have trouble shaking that mentality. And even for some of you whose kids are gluten-free, a little bit might be okay. But if you're following a strict gluten-free diet because of celiac disease or another condition, a little is not okay.

> *"My mother-in-law absolutely refuses to have any part of a discussion about celiac disease. She thinks we're just being difficult when we explain the limitations of the diet, and has called us 'overprotective.' She has the whole family thinking we're blowing things way out of proportion and exaggerating Emily's condition. It's really frustrating."*
>
> —David L.

If you're known to exaggerate about other things, it's likely that people will think you're exaggerating when you tell them your child can't have even one molecule of gluten. Remember the old story of the boy who cried "wolf"? Well, this is when it haunts you. Because if people think you're exaggerating, they're going to nod you off and then slip your son a cookie when you aren't looking.

Be sure to let them know that you're not exaggerating or blowing things out of proportion. If you have a reputation for stretching the facts, address this issue head on. Say something like, "I know I've exaggerated about things in the past, but this is extremely important, and I hope you'll take this seriously. Every molecule of gluten will, in fact, do damage to her, and it's crucial that everyone be aware of that."

Remind everyone that "double dipping" with the knife in margarine, jelly, peanut butter, and other containers contaminates it, even if they can't see the crumbs, and makes it off limits to your child (more about this in later chapters).

4. The "Just-Don't-Get-It" Category (Most Common)

> *"My best friend thinks she understands the diet, and even comments to me about how easy it is. But then I find that she's been feeding Cass rice with teriyaki sauce on it—and the teriyaki has wheat in it. I'm not mad—I realize this is a subtle and confusing part of the diet—but it's annoying because she thinks she gets it, but she doesn't."*
>
> —Tania T.

There are actually two breeds of the Just-Don't-Get-It species. There are the "I-gotcha-say-no-more-read-ya-loud-and-clear" Just-Don't-Get-Its, and the Admittedly Acquiescent Just-Don't-Get-Its.

The "I-gotcha-say-no-more-read-ya-loud-and-clear" variety is by far the most difficult to train, because they think they get it. But they don't. The telltale sign that you're dealing with this breed is the nod that comes too quickly. When you say, "She can't eat gluten," the person starts nodding ferociously as though they know exactly what you're talking about (also often accompanied by a smug grin, fingers pointed at you like a cocked gun, a wink, and a clucking of the tongue). It's not necessarily that they're trying to act like they know something they don't. It's just that they may think they know—but they don't.

Many people think they get it because they assume that gluten is something more familiar than it is—for instance, that gluten is the same thing as glucose; if it's kosher, it must be okay; or if it comes from a health food store and says "natural," it has to be safe.

I'm embarrassed to admit that my first day or two of learning the gluten-free life-style even I hung onto the hope that maybe "flour" was different from "wheat flour," and that as long as it didn't say, "wheat flour," it was okay. So these well-meaning folks think they're speaking our language, but they're not. Unless this is someone who spends a lot of time with your child and really needs to understand the complexities of the diet, give up. Say no more. They're a Just-Plain-Don't-Get-It, and the ferocious nodders are the toughest to teach.

The second breed of the Just-Don't-Get-It species is the Admittedly Acquiescent. These people know they're not going to get it, and they say nothing. They simply take all of the written information you give them, stack it neatly into a pile that they will surely never again touch, and listen quietly and without interruption to your "spiel." When you're finished, they offer no more than a blank stare and a vague acknowledgment that they know you were speaking and now you're finished.

Unfortunately, the Just-Don't-Get-It types are the most common. In most cases you have to just give up and pray they don't poison your child. It's best, when you have to entrust your child's meal to this type of person, to send something pre-made that can't be contaminated by utensils or dirty toasters.

How to Deal with Just-Don't-Get-It Friends and Family

Adjusting to the gluten-free lifestyle is difficult, at best. So it's understandable that you may feel resentment and anger when close friends and family fall into the Just-Don't-Get-It category. You want them to be able to support you, to help out—and instead, they make it more difficult. Not only do you have to deal with the diet without their help and understanding, but you have to watch out for the possibility that they will accidentally give your child gluten.

The fact is, they don't get it, and most likely, they never will. So deal with it; don't dwell on it. Give them a copy of this book or your GF products listing, and make sure you always provide them with gluten-free, pre-prepared meals and treats. Again, make sure your child understands her diet to the best of her ability so that she can politely refuse the cookie that her friend's mother sneaks her with loving intentions.

And how do you deal with the Cookie-Sneaker? It depends on how likely she is to really understand the diet. If you think there's hope, and that her mistake was based on loving intentions, gently point out to her that she gave her beloved grandchild gluten, and that you're sure she wouldn't want to cause her harm. But if she's destined to be a Just-Doesn't-Get-It for life, or if you suspect that the "accident" may have been intentional for some reason, then bite your tongue and hope that you can trust your child to make the right choice in the future.

Hiding Husbands: How to Pull Them Out of Their Caves

This section doesn't always pertain to husbands or men. Sometimes it's the other way around. But more often than not, I hear it from this perspective, so go with me here—realizing that I'm ultra-appreciative of the husbands and men who are understanding and supportive—and that I'm just trying to help with a common situation.

> *"When my doctor told me about Kylie's diagnosis, I turned to my husband for support; after all, I thought we were in this together. But he just shut down and won't deal with it at all—he hasn't even taken the time to learn what she can or can't eat. Now I feel even more alone than before."*
>
> —Jenny J.

All husbands, as the saying goes, are not created equal. It is therefore no surprise that their responses vary when a family decides to put a child on a gluten-free diet.

I realize that even to address this issue implies a sexist or stereotypical view of husbands/dads, and that in fact, many husbands/dads are reading this book in order to get a better handle on how to deal with their child's condition. Those husbands, and lucky wives of those husbands, may be excused from reading this section!

But the truth is that it is usually the moms who take on the primary responsibility for the care and feeding of their children. So, it is typically the moms who are first to suspect that something's wrong, the moms who begin the often arduous and usually frustrating process of seeking medical consultation, and, ultimately, the moms who have to take principal responsibility for learning to deal with the GF diet.

In my discussions with literally thousands of parents, I have found that the natural reaction for many dads is to run and hide. They don't, of course, literally run out of the room. And they may at first sound as though they're going to be very supportive—because they want to be supportive. But most of the time, they don't know how to start, and soon the mom has taken complete responsibility for learning the gluten-free diet.

It's important to realize that fathers want to be involved in this diet, but may not know how to offer their support. Since mothers are usually the ones who feed the kids, fathers may feel that they shouldn't step in and take over that responsibility. They may ask you, "Can Natalie eat this?" Don't be tempted to answer (even if just to yourself), "Of course not, Airhead! If you were more involved with her diet, you'd know that malt flavoring has gluten in it." No, not a good response at all.

Dads love their kids just as much as moms do, and for them to recognize that they may not even know what to feed their own child can be embarrassing. They may be scared that they will poison their own child with gluten. Rather than deal with these uncomfortable emotions, some men avoid the situation altogether, and refuse to become involved at all.

If the husband/dad in your family is making himself scarce and refusing to become involved, realize that it's up to you to give him a hand. You can help him to become more supportive and take more responsibility, which will be the ultimate win-win situation.

The first step is for you to help him learn about the gluten-free diet. The key is to teach him without him knowing that he's being taught. To "instruct" him may cause resentment and defensiveness, which will send him right back into that cave.

Instead, encourage him to become involved in the diet by asking him to plan a meal, or read labels at the grocery store. For some men, simply being involved in meal planning and preparation will be a new concept, not to mention the additional consideration of going gluten-free. The more he becomes involved, the more confidence he'll have in mastering the GF lifestyle, and the more active role he will take in your child's diet.

Remember to be supportive and kind. You both have interesting new challenges and issues ahead, and it's important that you deal with them in a cohesive, constructive, positive manner. Most importantly, remember that you have an audience—your kids are taking note.

Relatives in Denial: It's Not **My** Gene!

"When Tarryn was diagnosed, it occurred to us that several people on my wife's side of the family have 'stomach problems.' Now that we know what to look for, they all seem pretty classic celiac to us. Yet not a single one will get tested. They complain about 'irritable bowel syndrome' or a 'wheat allergy,' and we try to explain that they could have celiac disease, and they should be tested. But they just won't."

—Tom B.

When you talk with family members you may hear something along the lines of, "Well, she didn't get it from me!" Sometimes these are the same family members who suffer from "irritable bowel syndrome," have relatives who have had colon cancer, and find that they feel better when they avoid certain foods, such as beer or bread. But they definitely don't have celiac disease, no siree.

This denial may occur even if it's not celiac disease you're dealing with. Any condition that has a genetic component is likely to cause relatives to get a little squeamish. Not only do they not want to be blamed for making a genetic contribution, but they don't want to consider the fact that they or their children may be genetically predisposed.

The truth is that celiac disease, like many conditions, is inherited; the genes came from someone in your child's biological family. Recent studies of relatives of people diagnosed with celiac disease revealed that more than 20 percent of the relatives who showed no symptoms whatsoever tested positive for celiac disease.

It is imperative that close relatives of your child with celiac disease be tested, even if there is no evidence of a disorder. The overall familial prevalence of celiac disease is estimated to be approximately 10 to 30 percent in first-degree relatives of a diagnosed celiac. First-degree relatives include the parents, siblings, and children.

You can gently remind them of the consequences to people who have celiac disease and continue to eat gluten: They may be riddled with symptoms that don't always appear to be related, such as headaches (including migraines), fatigue, depression and anxiety, and even infertility. Furthermore, research indicates that they may be 40 to 100 times more likely to develop intestinal lymphoma (cancer); and they may develop myriad medical problems, including anemia, osteoporosis, and malnutrition. They will also likely experience gastrointestinal discomfort that they may mistakenly attribute to lactose intolerance, irritable bowel syndrome, stress, or gas.

See Chapter 22 for more information on familial incidence, genetics, and testing.

Discuss It Discreetly—Remember, Kids Have Ears, Too

People will ask you about your child's condition. They're curious, and there's nothing wrong with that. Don't feel offended or intruded upon because people ask why your child is politely refusing the birthday cake or team snack. Don't whisper or act ashamed; but at the same time, you don't need to tell everybody that your child has a special diet. Information should be distributed on a need-to-know basis. There are also varying amounts of information people might need to know. Always remember that your child is listening, so be careful how you phrase the information. You need to be accurate (don't call celiac disease an allergy!). But

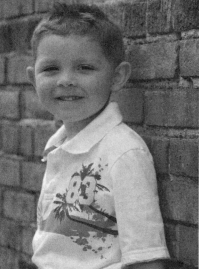

you don't want to make it sound as if it's a burden for you, either (until your child is out of the room—then you can dump on your closest friends).

You may want to prepare yourself early on so that you're not caught off-guard when someone asks. Depending upon the situation, the answer can be brief and factual, or lengthy and emotional. Here are a few conversation guides and some suggestions for different responses based on who you are talking to and their need-to-know rating:

◆ The really quick, you-probably-don't-really-care-anyway-but-I-feel-I-need-to-explain response. This is best used when the waitress asks, "What? No bun on the burger?" as though you've just asked for fried worms in your salad. You could choose just to say, "That's right—she doesn't like the bun." But if you say that, chances are good that the waitress will just grab a pre-prepared burger and pluck the bun off. That's not good enough for a child on a strict gluten-free diet. A better response could be, "She can't eat wheat and other things, so she can't eat the bun. It's also important that the bun never touch the burger patty." Or say something equally benign that will get the point across. (There are more tips for talking with restaurant staff in Chapter 18.)

◆ The response for acquaintances who are genuinely curious, but don't want to hear your life's story. How far you take it is best gauged by how much they seem to be "getting" as you explain it, but a good start is to say, "She has a condition called (fill in the blank). It requires that she be on a restricted diet—no gluten." Chances are at this point, they'll have questions: What is gluten? How did you find out she had it? Is it really rare? Will she outgrow it? Base your response from here on the questions you get.

◆ Friends—that's what they're there for. If you're talking with your best friend, get it off your chest. Let him or her know the gluten-free diet can be difficult. Frustrating. You get mad at your friends who don't get it. You get mad at your friends who have it so easy. You have enough stress in your life without having to deal with a restricted and some-times-difficult diet. When you're done, you'll feel better. Then you can get on with raising your happy, healthy gluten-free kid.

11

Making Your Kitchen a Gluten-Free Safety Zone

"I thought we were being pretty good about the diet. Then I realized we were using the same colander to drain my daughter's gluten-free pasta as we were using to drain the regular pasta. How careful should we be when preparing food in the kitchen?"

—Sandra-Marie G.

Making sure you stock up on gluten-free foods is crucial. But what do you do with those foods once you get them home? Have you taken a close look at your kitchen lately? You're going to have to. You might as well face it—the days of using one knife to spread anything on toast are toast. In fact, if you are making both gluten-containing and gluten-free peanut butter and jelly sandwiches, it is a four-knife process! (I explain in detail when I describe the "gob drop" later in this chapter.)

If you're eliminating casein or other allergens as well as gluten, it's even more of a challenge to create a safety zone in your kitchen. Cooking can be daunting enough with our busy schedules, but toss on top of that a limited diet and concerns about contamination, and it can seem overwhelming at first. Hang in there—this chapter will help you confront your cooking conundrums and create meals the entire family will enjoy.

The rules contained in this chapter—and in fact throughout this book—pertain to casein and other ingredients you need to avoid as they do to gluten. Rather than clutter the book with duplicitous references to gluten, casein, and other allergens, you'll see references to gluten and how to create safe gluten-free zones in your kitchen and cooking areas. Just know that the rules are the same for avoiding casein (and others) as they are for avoiding gluten, even if casein and others aren't specifically called out.

The major problem in keeping a kitchen gluten-free is inherent in nearly any kitchen. Have you ever looked into someone's jelly jar? It's a sort of disgusting exercise, really, and may kill your appetite for ever eating at their house again. The point is that

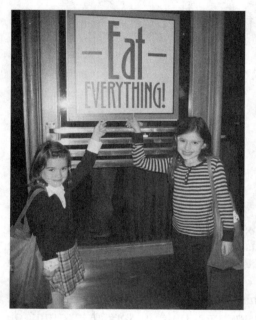

there are *crumbs*! Millions of gluten-containing, villi-blunting, diarrhea-inducing *crumbs* nesting comfortably in the jelly jar.

Unless your entire family is 100 percent gluten-free (and you therefore have a completely gluten-free kitchen), you need to be extremely careful about the possibility of cross-contamination. That means no sticking the knife back into the margarine container for "seconds" after spreading the first helping on toast. Any utensil that has touched gluten-containing food should not be used in the preparation of gluten-free foods. You can't stir the regular pasta and then use the same spoon to stir the GF stuff. You can't drain the pastas in the same colander, either, unless you wash it thoroughly. When you make a grilled cheese sandwich with regular bread, you can't use the same pan (until you wash it thoroughly) to make a GF sandwich.

It's not difficult to maintain a gluten-free-friendly kitchen, but it does take some getting used to and ongoing diligence. Make sure the entire family, even the very young kids and frequent visitors, understand the importance of it.

Tips for Keeping a GF-Friendly Kitchen
Spreadables

◆ Learn to do the "gob drop." No, it's not a new dance or video game. It's a method of scooping up a gob of margarine (or peanut butter, jelly, mayonnaise, or any other spread), and dropping it onto your slice of bread (or pancake—you get the idea). The key to a good gob drop is learning how *much* of a gob to grab. The beauty of the gob drop is that because the knife has not actually touched the bread, it's okay to reinsert it and go for another gob! But once you've used the knife to spread your gob, you cannot go back for more.

So why does it take four knives to make a peanut butter and jelly sandwich? Well, just imagine you're making two PB&Js: one with "regular" bread, and one with your really-delicious-because-you've-perfected-the-recipe gluten-free bread. Assume that you're using gluten-free peanut butter and jelly for both sandwiches. You start with the gluten-containing sandwich, and you use knife number-one for the peanut butter. After a carefully measured gob-drop, you are now ready to spread. But after the knife has touched the bread, it can no longer be used for *anything*! Not more peanut butter, not jelly—not *even* to finish making the "regular" sandwich! Because when that knife goes back into the jar, it is laden with gluten. You repeat the process with jelly, and before you know it, you've used several knives for just a couple of sandwiches!

Do you need to do the gob drop if you're dropping onto a gluten-free piece of bread (pancake, etc.)? You should. While the gluten-free crumbs won't cause a problem in terms of gluten contamination, the next time you make a sandwich they could cause you to stop and wonder whether the crumbs are gluten-containing or gluten-free. We have thrown away more than a few jars of mayonnaise because we didn't know for sure.

◆ Buy separate "spreadables." As an alternative to doing the "gob drop," you can keep separate containers for things that are easily contaminated, such as margarine, cream cheese, and jelly. It's safest to have separate containers, even if the margarine you use is GF. Mark the containers "GF only," and make sure they're used only for gluten-free food preparation.

Utensils

◆ Have separate colanders. Pasta leaves a residue, and is therefore very difficult to remove completely. It's a good idea to have separate colanders: one for gluten-free pastas, and one for gluten-containing pastas. (Of course you could drain the gluten-free pasta first, and make sure you wash it thoroughly after you drain gluten-containing pasta in it.) Because you might want to make two types of pasta on spaghetti night—one with gluten and one without—it's easiest to make them at the same time and use two separate colanders. If you have more than one, it's a good idea to dedicate one of them to the gluten-free pastas, and then mark them with a permanent marker so that there will never be any question which colander is used for which type of pasta.

◆ It goes both ways. When separating utensils and other items used in the kitchen, remember that it's just as important to keep gluten-free foods *out* of the "gluten-only" containers as it is to keep gluten-containing foods out of the gluten-free containers. In other words, it's obvious that you don't want to put gluten-containing pasta into a gluten-free colander. But sometimes people forget that putting gluten-free pasta into a colander dedicated for "regular" pasta is just as bad! The gluten residue on the colander contaminates the GF pasta, defeating the purpose of separating the utensils in the first place.

◆ Use lots of aluminum foil. To ensure that gluten-free food remains uncontaminated, use aluminum foil for any cooking you do on a cookie sheet, or any other surface, for that matter. If you prefer to cook directly on the sheet, make sure you designate one for gluten-free purposes, keep it in a separate area, if possible, and never use it with gluten-containing food.

Making and Toasting Bread

◆ Buy a breadmaker. Even if you love to bake, I suggest buying a breadmaker, because you will be making a lot of bread and it will make your life easier when you're out of time and energy. Gluten-free dough is far heavier than "regular" dough, so you'll need to do some research to find a breadmaker that can accommodate the heavier consistency. Look for the models with the greatest horsepower and large mixing paddles. I'm not saying it's absolutely *necessary* to buy a breadmaker. Many mixes turn out well without one, and the bakers amongst you may not need one either. But breadmakers can help if you're short on time, or if the kids make their own bread. If you're going casein-free too, you'll be happy to find several gluten-free/casein-free bread mixes available that you can make quickly in a breadmaker.

◆ While you're at it, buy a bread slicer. Bread slicers can be found near the breadmakers at most stores that carry household items. The loaf of bread fits inside the slicer, which has slits every ¾" or so. The slicer comes with an electric knife, which you insert into the slits as you cut. It slices the bread in even slices and makes it look just like "regular" bread. As you know, how it *looks* is every bit as important as how it *tastes* to a child!

◆ Have separate toasters or toaster ovens. Once a "regular" piece of bread touches the grill of a toaster or toaster oven, the grill is contaminated, and you should not use that same toaster or toaster oven for GF bread (unless everyone in your family is very good about wiping off the toaster after gluten-containing bread has been used). If you have a four-slice toaster, you may be tempted to dedicate two of the slots for GF bread, leaving the other two slots for regular bread. Don't do it. Anyone who has wiped up around a toaster knows that toast practically *throws* its crumbs around. There is almost no way to pull a piece of regular bread out of one slot without dropping crumbs into another slot. Unless your kitchen is 100 percent gluten-free, there's really no way around it—you need separate toasters. Forget aesthetics and get out that permanent marker, clearly marking one "gluten-free" and the other "gluten only." That way even guests won't make a mistake.

Food Preparation

◆ Clean those crumbs! Remember to wipe up bread crumbs and other gluten-containing messes. All it takes is for someone to set a gluten-free sandwich on a plate that had a gluten-containing item on it, and the whole point of eating that gluten-free sandwich is for naught.

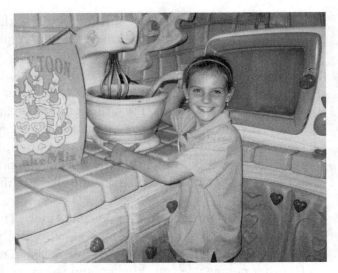

◆ Get in the habit of making the GF version first. If you're making a grilled cheese sandwich, make the GF version first. That way you can use the same pan (assuming it has a good nonstick finish and you clean it well) for both the gluten-free and the regular versions. While you're getting into new habits, you might as well get used to making more of the gluten-free version than you think you'll need. Otherwise, just as you finish cooking the heavily gluten-laden sandwich, your child with celiac disease will change his mind and decide that yes, he does in fact want another one. And then you get to wash the pan *two* more times!

◆ Order mixes. Thanks to greater availability and some large manufacturers producing more GF products, you can, if you choose, avoid specialty stores, doing most of your shopping at a regular grocery store. However, there are some products that you might need to buy online if you can't find them locally. These include mixes for bread, pizza dough crust, pancakes, cakes, cookies, brownies, and muffins. You'll appreciate that stash of cake mixes when you suddenly realize that one of your child's classmates is having a birthday party at school!

◆ Be creative. Get in the habit of thinking, "How can I make that gluten-free" when you see a delicious recipe or meal. There are suggestions for being especially creative in Chapter 13.

Food Storage

◆ Try to separate the GF foods in the pantry and refrigerator. By dedicating shelves or drawers to gluten-free (and casein-free if your child avoids casein) products, you accomplish a few things. You decrease the chance that a guest or babysitter will accidentally give your child something with gluten. In addition, if guests or babysitters have questions about whether or not a food is safe, by having gluten-free foods in designated areas, you eliminate any question. Maybe most importantly, you create the perception that there are lots of things your child can eat. Sometimes when children look in a pantry, they tend to see so many foods that they *can't* have that they have trouble seeing the things they *can* eat. This can be really disheartening for them. But when they see shelves loaded with gluten-free items—even if they're not treats, but just mixes, pasta, and other "staples," they realize that there are lots of things they can eat.

◆ Make a special "GF Treats" area. Keep a drawer or cupboard that is designated especially for your gluten-free child, and make sure it's filled with all sorts of great treats. It's important to have an area that he sees *filled* with fun foods that he can eat—even if you have to make him wait until after dinner! It's not enough just to have the treats on hand, mixed with all the other gluten-containing treats. Kids tend to look at the entire picture, and see "nothing" that they can eat.

◆ Buy small, brightly colored removable labels. These work well for sticking on plastic ware used to store leftovers. You can write your child's name or just "GF" (or "GF/CF") on the label, or simply have a designated "GF color" for food containers. (If other people use your kitchen and feed your kids, a "GF color" may not be clear enough. If that's the case, you should write your child's name or "GF" on the label.)

When Guests Visit

Okay, so you've finally gotten the routine down, and even your two-year-old has perfected the gob drop. But now you have a houseful of guests coming for Thanksgiving. Personally, I love a "mi casa es su casa" environment. We frequently have people staying with us, and they're encouraged to help themselves to anything in the fridge.

Accommodating, yes. But visiting guests who help themselves to the fridge will be your greatest challenge in keeping a GF-friendly kitchen.

If the guests are regulars, it's important to initially explain in detail how critical it is to keep the kitchen GF-friendly. Chances are they are already well aware of your child's condition, but the extent of their understanding will vary, depending upon whose friend it is, how old they are, and how tuned-in they are to the situation. Whether they understand or not, it is crucial to teach all guests that there is never any double-dipping in the spreadables. If your toasters and utensils are well marked, it should be clear what can and can't be used for food preparation, but call it to their attention in the beginning, just in case. You'll have to watch closely at first, and even years later you'll find your blood pressure increases every time guests are cooking in your kitchen.

If the guests are not regulars, you need to decide how much information to give them. Gauge their interest level, their ability to thoroughly understand, how long they're staying, and how likely they are to use the kitchen. One helpful trick is to buy small tubs of the spreadables your child is most likely to need for the duration of the visit—margarine, peanut butter, cream cheese, mayo. Mark his containers clearly with his name followed by the word "ONLY!" and threatening pictures of what will happen to anyone else who uses it. Make sure that your child eats only from those containers during the visit.

Try to teach your visitors the gob drop. Some will get it, but some just can't resist sticking the knife back into the container. Work with them, and try to educate them in a firm but friendly way, but remember to use the dedicated gluten-free spreadables for your child. When the guests have gone, the safest option is to toss the "community containers" and start with new ones. Consider it part of the cost of entertaining.

Most of the time, you'll find it's easier just to do all the meal preparation and serving yourself. But don't fall into that trap. Guests *like* to help, and you don't want to make them feel awkward. Give them something to do that won't involve a risk of cross-contamination. Have them wash the veggies or slice the meat, and prepare yourself for the fact that there probably will be mistakes, and that life will go on.

12

Shopping:
Is There More to Life Than Fritos?

"Off I went—boldly going where it seemed no one else had ever gone—my first shopping trip in search of gluten-free goodies. My son was begging for crackers, so I started in the cracker aisle, trying to find one without gluten. You know, not one single package had 'gluten' in the ingredients. I was delighted! What a breeze this was going to be!"

—Danna Korn

The day Tyler was diagnosed with celiac disease I was paralyzed with fear—terrified to feed my own child! After pulling myself together and remembering that my bloated-belly toddler needed me to be strong for him (and was starving after a long day at the hospital), I armed myself with the blue sheet of forbidden ingredients that I had gotten from the less-than-helpful hospital dietitian, and headed to my neighborhood grocery store.

My son was begging for crackers, so I started in the cracker aisle, trying to find one without gluten. Hmmm. You know, not one single package had "gluten" in the ingredients. I was delighted! What a breeze this was going to be! But then I checked my list again—"flour." My heart sank. Could it possibly be by some grace of God that *flour* is different from *wheat flour*? After all, the ingredients label doesn't *say* "wheat flour," it just says "flour." It was hopeful and naïve thinking, I knew.

On with the search for a cracker that Tyler could eat. It only takes a few hours of dealing with the gluten-free diet to know there's no point in even going *down* the cracker aisle, but I was in my infancy of gluten-free(dom), and thought maybe some of the "rice crackers" would be okay. Flour in everything. I gave up and headed to the bread aisle. Yeah, I don't need to tell you how that turned out. That was, after all, 1991.

By now we were well into the second hour of "shopping," with a completely empty cart. My son and I were both crying—he because he was hungry and bored, and I because I couldn't have been sadder or more frustrated. And this was only the beginning.

As we started to leave, I passed through the chips aisle and happened to pick up a bag of Fritos. What? No flour? I checked the huge list of forbidden additives, and none were found in the ingredients listing on this precious bag of Fritos! My sadness turned to relief and gratitude. I grabbed four bags and headed for the check-out stand. At least he wouldn't starve. But would there be life after Fritos?

Can You Ever Do Most of Your Shopping at a "Regular" Grocery Store Again?

Many parents who are new to the idea of putting their kids on a GF diet fear that they will have to do all of their shopping in expensive and inconvenient health food stores. Well, stop worrying about taking out that third mortgage just to pay the food bill. Because you *can* do most of your shopping at a regular grocery store, and it's really not that hard to do, once you figure out a family menu plan that works for you. You can even buy generic foods, if you put a little effort into it. Yes, you might still need to head to a natural foods store from time to time, and you might even want to buy some foods online—but 95 percent of your shopping can be done at your neighborhood grocery store.

> "I figure my days of shopping at the local grocery store are history. I'm assuming I'll have to do all of my shopping at a health food store or by mail—that's so expensive and inconvenient!"
>
> —Charlanne O.

Start by stocking up on gluten-free staples. Some will be more expensive, but the peace of mind is well worth the money.

Gluten-Free Staples to Stock Up On

Some brands of the following staple items contain gluten, and others don't. In fact, there are many staples that rarely, if ever, contain gluten. But even for those that usually do contain gluten (e.g., soy sauce), with a little homework (calls to manufacturers, label reading, and/or gluten-free shopping guides), it's easy to find the following "staple items" in any major grocery chain, and there are plenty of casein-free alternatives for those going casein-free, too.

- mayonnaise
- ketchup
- mustard
- gluten-free soy sauce
- gluten-free teriyaki sauce
- salad dressings
- margarine/butter
- sugar
- brown sugar
- cornstarch
- nonstick sprays
- yogurt
- milk
- hot cocoa
- marshmallows
- cheese
- chili
- chicken stock
- soups

Develop a List of Safe Products Your Child Likes

As you try different brands and types of foods, create a product listing of gluten-free foods your child likes. Keep it neatly organized so that when you need the information, it's there. You may even want to have two copies, each in a three-ring binder. You can keep one in the pantry and one in the car (so that you can check on particular products if you're at the grocery store or a restaurant and the need arises). If you're tech-savvy, keep the list on your phone. There are even new apps that have databases of GF foods for smart phones. (See www.clanthompson.com for more on the new apps!)

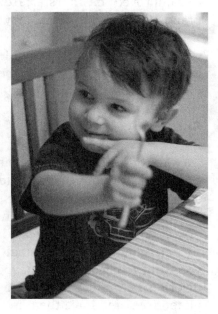

If you want to generate your own list, give yourself a head start by going to the product listings at manufacturers' websites. There are some phenomenal sites now! And remember, just because an item is *not* on a published gluten-free list does *not* mean it has gluten in it. Keep digging to be sure.

- ***Date your products list.*** Whether you make your own list as a result of calls to manufacturers or are using lists received from companies, date them! Ingredients change, and you should check frequently to make sure the products are still gluten-free.

- ◆ *Call manufacturers.* Get in the habit of calling every toll-free number you can find on the side of a box. It doesn't matter whether the product appears to be gluten-free or not—it can be a box of saltines, for that matter. But call to ask if they have a list of their gluten-free products. You'll be pleasantly surprised at how many food distributors and manufacturers are very knowledgeable about gluten.
- ◆ *Get out that permanent marker.* It's a good idea to mark "GF" in permanent marker directly on the product labels when you learn they're gluten-free. This will avoid any questions, especially if other people are feeding your kids.
- ◆ *Save labels of safe foods for a month or two.* In the beginning, before you're *really* organized, it can be very helpful to save the labels of products that you discover are gluten-free. Keep them in a large zip-seal bag, and take them to the grocery store with you, just in case you have trouble remembering which items are safe. Of course, after a few months the safe products will be etched in your brain!

Beware of "New and Improved"

Most consumers get excited when they see the words "new and improved." Not us. Sure, it's usually just a marketing gimmick, but for people avoiding gluten, "new and improved" means "start from scratch" in ensuring that it's gluten-free. That trusty brand of gluten-free cereal may not be so gluten-free anymore.

Even without label changes, remember that just because a product is gluten-free today doesn't mean that it will be gluten-free tomorrow. Check labels frequently for ingredient changes, and call the manufacturers often to make sure that their sources and ingredients are still gluten-free.

Buying Generics

Yes, it's even possible to buy gluten-free generic products. The first thing to do is contact the corporate headquarters for the chain of stores you prefer, and ask if they have a list of their gluten-free products. These days, chances are pretty good that you'll score! Some major grocery chains even have a list of their generic GF products on the Internet.

If your preferred stores don't have a list, you can dig a little to find the generics that are gluten-free. Start small, and be prepared. Pick four or five generic foods that you want to check into—maybe things that you want your child to eat or that were favorites before her diagnosis. Buy them, even not knowing whether or not they're gluten-free, and have them in front of you before you call. Call the corporate headquarters and work your way to their head nutritionist or quality assurance specialist. It's not always easy to find that person, but persevere, and you will get there.

Be nice! This person can be your very best friend, or can be lazy and give you the dreaded, "I don't know." But if you say that you realize you are asking a lot, but could they help you determine whether or not some of the foods are gluten-free, chances are they'll be receptive and cooperative.

Unfortunately, you can't just ask whether the products are gluten-free. Focus on the ingredients that are suspect—natural flavorings, for instance. Ask if they can find out what the source is: barley, corn, or another source. Usually they know that information right away. Go through all of the suspect ingredients until you have determined that the product is or is not gluten-free. If it is GF, make note of it, keep it in your binder, and be sure to check back often because ingredients, as you know, can change.

Shop Name Brands

Whether you're a brand-name shopper or not, kids usually are. They like to know that they're eating brands that all the other kids eat—but when they're on a gluten-free diet, that can present challenges. Don't be deterred. There are lots of great GF name-brand items out there now. Seek them out! Call the manufacturers and get a list of their gluten-free goodies, and make sure to have them on hand. Believe it or not, for some kids and in some cases taste takes a back seat to branding. Don't feel you have to buy *everything* name-brand—but a few visible items like chips in the lunch box will go a long way in making your child feel better about her diet.

Menu Planning

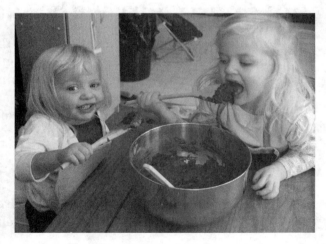

Regardless of your dietary issues, planning meals before you head to the store is always going to help you save time and money. When you have dietary restrictions, planning in advance is even more important. One of the most important things to do if you want to shop at a "regular" grocery store is to figure out several meals that your entire family enjoyed before embarking upon your gluten-free lifestyle, and revise them to be gluten-free. For instance, if your family enjoys burritos made with flour tortillas, improvise with corn tortillas. If your family likes ranch dressing but the dressing you use has gluten in it, find one that is gluten-free and switch. The next chapter will specifically outline suggested menu ideas.

Be sure to plan ahead. Before shopping, make sure you know what meals you want to prepare that week. Not only will that allow you the opportunity to make calls before you go to the store to determine if specific products are gluten-free, but it will help you decide where you need to shop.

Shopping at Health Food Stores or by Mail Order and Online

There are some staple gluten-free items you'll definitely want to have on hand, some of which aren't readily available in regular grocery stores yet (notice the optimistic "yet" comment!). For those, you'll want to check out your local health food store or pick them up online. The good news is that these days, most of these "staples" taste incredible! You almost can't go wrong with the wonderful mixes available today. It's a good idea to stock up on them, so that when you need them they're there. These items include:

- ◆ bread mix (to be made with or without a breadmaker),
- ◆ pizza dough crust mix and ready-made pizza crusts,
- ◆ pasta (all different shapes; kids love to have a variety),
- ◆ mixes for cookies, muffins, brownies, cakes,
- ◆ baking mix (to make a variety of baked goods),
- ◆ pancake/waffle mix, and
- ◆ ready-to-eat snacks, such as ice cream cones and pretzels.

Mixing It Up with Mixes

Don't feel guilty about using mixes rather than baking from scratch. Ingredients for gluten-free baked goods—such as xanthan gum and the variety of different flours used—are very expensive. The cost usually turns out to be the same or even less (especially if you count all the really gross batches of breads and cookies you'll have to throw away if you're experimenting on your own) when you use mixes.

Another great thing about mixes is that they're easy enough for some kids to make themselves at an early age (or, with some adult supervision). Remember, keeping the kids involved in their food selection and preparation gives them a sense of control, and helps them feel good about their diet.

The best reason to stock up on and use mixes is that the mixes have come a *long* way! When my son was first diagnosed with celiac disease, there weren't any mixes

Brand-Name Baking Mixes

What names are more trustworthy for tasty mixes than Betty Crocker and Bisquick? I used to dream that someday there would be gluten-free Betty Crocker mixes on the shelves—and that just goes to show ya that dreams do come true! Today there are several varieties of GF Betty Crocker mixes, and Bisquick has even gone gluten-free! There are even more great General Mills gluten-free mixes and products to come in the future.

that we could buy for baked goods, so we had to make our baked goods from scratch. Once, when he was three, I worked all day in the kitchen perfecting a chocolate chip cookie recipe to the point where I thought it was just about palatable. I felt like June Cleaver, and was *so* excited to be able to offer Tyler and his three-year-old buddy, A.J., some cookies, fresh from the oven—an act most moms take for granted.

Beaming, I set the plate in front of them and watched carefully for their reactions. Tyler took his cookie first. His eyes lit up, and he said, "Yummy cookie, Mommy!" A.J. ran for the nearest trash can and spat for a good five minutes.

If you prefer to grind your own rice flour and bake from scratch, you have my respect and admiration. But if you're limited on time, or just don't have the desire to bake from scratch every time, give the mixes a try.

Get Used to Stocking Up

Because there are some items that aren't as readily available, it's a good idea to stock up on those products. It's also a good idea to stock up on your child's favorites when you encounter them. Especially good brands or flavors of cereal, crackers, pasta, mixes, pretzels, and other difficult-to-find items are welcome sights in the pantry when you're caught short on menu ideas.

13

The Chapter You've Been Waiting For:
Menu and Snack Ideas!

"Hunter really misses chicken fingers, fish sticks, corn dogs, and other things he can't have anymore. I'm really not much of a cook and can't figure out how to make these things without gluten."

—Danielle V.

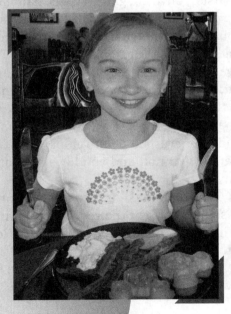

For those of you who didn't jump right to this chapter, you've learned to work through some tough emotions, decipher confusing labels, and work your way through the gluten-free shopping adventures. But I know—feeding your hungry kid is, after all, what this book is all about! So let's get to it with some menu and snack ideas.

I don't do recipes in this book. For one thing, there are several excellent cookbooks out there that are loaded with terrific gluten-free recipes. Many of the recipes for baked goods that you'll find in those cookbooks require rice, tapioca, potato, or other gluten-free flours, and other ingredients you may not usually use, such as xanthan or guar gum. Having tried a number of those recipes (and written some gluten-free cookbooks of my own), I can tell you that recipes you'll find are delicious, and you most definitely will want some of those cookbooks on hand.

But there are plenty of times when you just don't want to have to mix a bunch of flours, or pay ludicrous amounts of money for ingredients like xanthan gum. That's what this chapter is about—learning to be a creative cook in a gluten-free sort of way.

This chapter will spark some ideas so that you can put together quick snacks and easy meals that your child will enjoy. Because they're simple, common-sense ideas, you'll be able to modify dishes quickly and easily that your entire family enjoys.

Getting Creative Is Easy!

The most important thing about cooking from now on is to *be creative*. Don't despair, thinking that your child will never again enjoy chicken nuggets. Grab some gluten-free flour—it really doesn't matter what kind—and roll the chicken in it. A bunch of oil and a big mess later, you have chicken nuggets! Thought doughnuts were a thing of the past? Nope. Buy a doughnut maker, use any gluten-free muffin or cake mix you have lying around, and voila! Doughnuts! Need a pie crust? Crush some gluten-free cookies, add some margarine, and push it into a pie tin.

Really, almost anything can be modified to be gluten-free, and usually it's not too tough to do so. (The exceptions are for breads, homemade pastas, cookies, cakes, and muffins. You'll be most successful using a mix or a gluten-free recipe for these.)

If you want to make an old family favorite but it isn't gluten-free, work with it. To illustrate how easy it is to adapt a recipe to be gluten-free, I just now opened a cookbook (*Weight Watchers Quick Meals*) and landed on a page with a recipe for Crunchy Garlic-Broiled Halibut. Ingredients include parsley, olive oil, garlic cloves, halibut steaks, and bread crumbs. Substitute crunched-up potato chips for the bread crumbs, and you have yourself a gluten-free version that probably tastes even better than the original.

Feel like making a fancy gourmet dish like chicken cordon bleu? Take chicken breasts, flatten them out (you may want to pound them to make them more tender), and put a dab of butter or sour cream, slivers of ham, and some spices in the middle. Then roll the chicken breast around the goodies in the middle so you have a "ball." Roll that in any gluten-free mix you have in the house (it really doesn't matter if it's a bread mix, pancake, or even muffin mix), or crushed potato chips. Then bake or deep fry, depending upon whether it's "diet day" or not, and you have a great meal that's probably too gourmet for your kids anyway.

Think ahead. If you're making GF bread, make an extra batch of dough and put it in the fridge or freezer. Then, someday when the rest of the family is having bread or rolls with dinner, pull out a handful of dough and roll it into a long "snake" or stick, or drop a few spoonfuls into muffin tins. You may want to drizzle a little butter on top for an added treat. Then pop them in the oven, and make fresh-baked bread sticks or biscuits. The house will smell great, and you'll feel like Gluten-Free Mom of the Year!

So go ahead . . . live "la vida loca"—get wild, crazy, and *creative*!

Homemade "Hamburger Helper"

Maybe someday Hamburger Helper will have a gluten-free version, but for now, while it's one of America's favorite meals, it's off-limits for anyone who's gluten free. But with a little experimentation and creativity, you can come up with recipes for any of the convenience foods your child craves, including Hamburger Helper. Here's an idea of how to make a homemade version that's almost as hassle-free as the name brand.

- ◆ Cook 1 lb. hamburger or ground turkey. Drain fat.
- ◆ Add taco seasoning packet (many brands available in grocery stores are gluten-free) or salsa.
- ◆ In a separate pot, boil about two cups gluten-free pasta (elbows or fun shapes are best). Drain when completely cooked.
- ◆ Add pasta to the hamburger mixture.
- ◆ Sprinkle cheese or cheese substitute on top.

Substitution Ideas for Turning Gluten into Gluten-Free

For those of you eliminating casein too, there are lots of milk and dairy substitutes available. Since they're relatively straightforward (e.g., milk substitute, cheese substitute), this section focuses more on the gluten-free substitutions you can make in creating a gluten-free meal.

If a recipe calls for . . .

- ◆ *Soy sauce:* use gluten-free soy sauce (at least a couple of national brands can be found at most major grocery stores) or Bragg's Amino Acids (similar to soy sauce).
- ◆ *Thickening with flour:* use cornstarch, arrowroot flour, or a GF bread mix (or any other GF mix) you have handy.
- ◆ *Coating with flour or bread crumbs* (to fry or sauté): coat with a gluten-free bread mix, cornmeal, or crushed potato chips.
- ◆ *Croutons:* cut some gluten-free bread into cubes, and deep fry or even pan fry in butter.
- ◆ *Pie crust:* crush up old gluten-free cookies or cereal, mix with melted butter, and press into a pie tin.
- ◆ *Pasta:* use gluten-free pasta (usually the sauce for toppings is gluten-free).
- ◆ *Flour tortillas:* use corn tortillas, or use rice wraps found in Asian markets or the Asian food section of grocery stores.
- ◆ *Pasta pieces* (as in rice pilaf, for instance): use crumbled pieces of gluten-free pasta.

◆ *Crackers:* use rice crackers or Savory Thins.
◆ *Bun* (for hamburgers or sandwiches): use gluten-free bread, corn tortilla, or lettuce wrap.
◆ *Sauce:* try salsa, melted cheese, or mayonnaise mixed with ketchup.
◆ *Thickener for sweets:* use dry pudding mix (several gluten-free varieties are available in the stores), or cornstarch and sugar.

Quick Meal Ideas

Okay, you're ready to cook, or at least to prepare some quick treats! Here are some menu-planning ideas to get you going. Note that I refer to a number of products that can be gluten-free or not (e.g., yogurt, soy sauce, cream cheese, etc.). Make sure that you check the ingredients for each of these foods.

Breakfast

◆ Eggs, cooked any way your child will eat (hey, moms and dads can't be picky!)
◆ Egg in a basket
  ➤ Butter both sides of a piece of gluten-free bread. Tear a hole in it, fry it in a frying pan, and drop an egg in the hole. Flip when the cooked side is golden brown. Cook until the other side is golden brown, too.
◆ Fruit
  ➤ It's fun to dig out a scoop of kiwi, pear, or cantaloupe and put a spoonful of yogurt in it.
◆ Toast (gluten-free)
  ➤ Remember, the breadmaker and slicer are lifesavers!
◆ Cereal
◆ As you're aware, many cereals have malt flavoring and are off-limits. But some big manufacturers are starting to change that, and GF cereals are more widely available on the shelves now. There are also lots of specialty brands that even regular grocery stores sell. Just watch for malt flavoring, oats, and of course any other gluten-containing ingredients.
◆ Quesadillas (a warm tortilla with melted cheese inside)—Use corn tortillas, of course.
◆ Bacon
  ➤ There are several gluten-free brands available at any grocery store.
◆ Sausage
  ➤ There are several gluten-free brands available at any grocery store.
◆ Yogurt

◆ Smoothie
  ➤ Fruit blended in blender with orange juice, milk, or ice cream. I usually try to dump some protein powder in there when the kids aren't looking.
◆ Instant breakfast
  ➤ There are commercial brands that are gluten-free; you should check status (the most common gluten-containing ingredient you'll find in these is malt).
◆ Grits or rice cereal, served with butter, cinnamon-sugar, or syrup on top.
◆ French toast (made from slices of gluten-free bread)
◆ Pancakes
  ➤ There are several excellent gluten-free pancake mixes available by mail. Many health food stores sell gluten-free pancake/waffle mixes.
◆ Waffles
  ➤ There are several good GF mixes, and some excellent pre-made GF freezer waffles that you just warm in a toaster or toaster oven. The freezer waffles can be found in health food stores, or even in national grocery chains in the health food section.

Lunch

◆ Sandwiches (made with gluten-free bread)
  ➤ Peanut butter and jelly, cucumber and cream cheese, ham, cheese—the only thing limiting your options (besides gluten) is your creativity!
◆ Waffle sandwich
  ➤ If you don't have any gluten-free bread handy, use a frozen GF waffle (toast it first) instead.
◆ Tamales or taquitos
  ➤ There are several commercial GF brands sold at grocery stores (made with corn).
◆ Quesadillas
  ➤ Corn tortilla, of course.
◆ Fruit
◆ Hot dogs (gluten-free) (no bun)
  ➤ There are several commercial gluten-free brands sold in grocery stores.
  ➤ For a bun, try wrapping a corn tortilla around the hot dog, then heating in a microwave. The juices from the hot dog will steam the tortilla.
◆ Hamburger (no bun)

- ◆ Nachos
  - ➤ Corn tortilla chips with cheese melted on them. Feel free to add chicken, beef, veggies, beans, or any other leftovers you have.
- ◆ Tuna and mayonnaise on GF toast or GF crackers
- ◆ Tuna melt
- ◆ Grilled cheese sandwich
- ◆ Grilled chicken on a GF bun or with lettuce wrap
- ◆ Macaroni and cheese
  - ➤ You can either buy gluten-free pasta and melt your own cheese on it, or check health food stores for gluten-free varieties of "macaroni and cheese" in a box that are similar to the gluten-containing commercial brands.
- ◆ Pizza
  - ➤ You can either make your own crust from a cookbook recipe or mix, or put pizza "fixin's" on a corn tortilla or piece of gluten-free bread.
  - ➤ There are several online and mail-order companies that sell excellent pre-made pizza crusts; stock up and freeze them.
- ◆ Spaghetti with GF pasta (let your kids shape the meatballs)
- ◆ Cheese and GF crackers
- ◆ Hard-boiled eggs
- ◆ Baked beans (check the brand) and GF weenies or bacon
- ◆ Soup (travels well in a lunchbox in a small thermos)
- ◆ Quiche (crustless or with a crust made from GF Bisquick)
- ◆ Frittatas

Dinner

- ◆ Hamburger or turkey burger (no bun)
- ◆ Meatloaf
  - ➤ Put GF bread crumbs or crushed nonsweetened gluten-free cereal in if you have some available; otherwise do without and mix an egg, barbecue sauce, and the meat, then bake).
- ◆ Taco salad
  - ➤ Put corn tortilla chips on the bottom (they're the best part), salad, chicken or hamburger with taco spice, beans, grated cheese, and anything else you can think of. Top it with your favorite salad dressing or salsa.
- ◆ Spaghetti or other pasta (gluten-free)
  - ➤ Several commercial brands of spaghetti sauce are gluten-free.
  - ➤ Make meatballs (no breading, of course) to go on top.
- ◆ Macaroni and cheese (as described under Lunch)
- ◆ Creamed tuna on toast

➤ Mix tuna, cream, a dab of butter, and a teaspoon of corn starch to thicken it; then serve over gluten-free toast.
◆ Tamales
◆ Taquitos
◆ Quesadillas (made with corn tortillas)
◆ Tacos
   ➤ Most hard shells at the store are gluten-free. You may also use corn tortillas raw or deep fried in oil.
◆ Barbecued or steamed vegetables
◆ Soup
   ➤ You can find lots of gluten-free soups in regular grocery stores these days. But you can also get creative and make your own soups using a gluten-free chicken broth for the base, or one of the several gluten-free brands of bouillon.
◆ Fish, shrimp, or any other favorite from the sea (no breading, but marinated in a gluten-free sauce and grilled or broiled is delicious and nutritious!).
◆ Pizza
   ➤ We make a few GF crusts at a time and freeze them, so that we can pull them out and put sauce, cheese, pepperoni, and anything else we want on them for a quick pizza.
   ➤ Another quick option is to use gluten-free bread or a corn tortilla as the "crust," and add the toppings.
◆ Hot dogs (gluten-free)
◆ Shish kebobs
◆ Tuna melt
◆ Chinese chicken salad
   ➤ Use tortilla chips, rice crackers, or maifun rice (from Asian market) for crunchies.
◆ Teriyaki chicken
   ➤ Most grocery stores carry gluten-free teriyaki, although it can be difficult to find at first.
◆ Polska Kielbasa
   ➤ There are gluten-free brands in the grocery stores.
◆ Steak or other favorite meat
◆ Cabbage rolls
   ➤ Inside the roll you can put hamburger meat, vegetables, rice, or any combination thereof.
◆ Chili
◆ Chicken nuggets (or you can use fish and make fish sticks)
   ➤ Cut the chicken or fish into nuggets or sticks. Coat with anything you have handy: a bread or pancake mix, or barbecued potato chips. Fry in oil or bake.

- ◆ "Wraps"
  - ➤ Use corn tortillas to wrap just about anything. Salad with salad dressing, beans and rice, avocado and turkey . . . get creative!
  - ➤ Use rice wrappers, found in Asian markets, or even the Asian foods section of your grocery store. They can be used cold, as a soft wrap, or deep fried into a crunchy wrap like on a spring roll.

Explore New Cuisines

Keep your eyes open for gluten-free foods from other countries that you may not have tried before. One day we were eating at a Thai restaurant, and noticed many "rice wrap" dishes. Some of the wraps were cold and uncooked; others were deep fried to a crispy crunch. We asked to see the package for the rice wrappers, and were delighted to discover that they were 100 percent rice flour, and apparently gluten-free. We jotted down the name of the manufacturer and distribution company, called to confirm their gluten-free status, and asked where they distributed these wrappers in our area. Within minutes, we had the names of several Asian markets and grocery stores in our area that carried them.

Side Dishes

- ◆ Rice
  - ➤ Don't be afraid to jazz it up. There are several pre-packaged Spanish rices (and other flavors) available at the store, or you can make your own. You can also put coconut milk in it to make it creamy.
- ◆ Potatoes
  - ➤ Cut new potatoes into small pieces and fry them in whatever seasonings you have available, bake your own French fries, or make mashed potatoes sometime other than Thanksgiving or Christmas.
  - ➤ Some brands of boxed "potato buds" are gluten-free.
  - ➤ Make twice-baked potatoes. (Cut open baked potatoes, mix the "insides" with margarine, cheese, bacon, and/or chives; put back in and bake with cheese on top)
  - ➤ Potato salad
- ◆ Quinoa (one of my favorite foods!)
- ◆ Corn bread or corn muffins (check that the recipe or mix is GF)
- ◆ Croutons for salad or soup
  - ➤ Either use the gluten-free bread you have to make these (cut in cubes, deep fry, roll in parmesan cheese or seasonings), or use tortilla chips as croutons.
- ◆ Refried beans
- ◆ Salad

- Vegetables, barbecued or almost any way you like them
- Applesauce

Snacks

> *"Our family is in the car a lot, and I have a hard time coming up with easy, healthy snacks that travel well.*
>
> —Theresa M.

Since there aren't many packaged "convenience" foods that are gluten-free, you sometimes need to get more creative. The following snacks are fun and easy.

- Chips
  - There are *many* flavors of gluten-free chips available at grocery stores! See Chapter 15 for some specific brands.
- String cheese
- Fried string cheese (roll string cheese in any gluten-free flour you have available and fry it up)
- Taquitos, quesadillas, tacos, tamales (made with corn tortillas)
- Nachos
- Corn Nuts
- Raisins and other dried fruit
- Chex "mix" (Chex now comes in several varieties that are gluten-free, but you'll need to make your own Chex "mix," as the kind that comes pre-packaged contains gluten)
- Popcorn
- Cheese cubes with toothpicks in them (not for the little ones!) and rice crackers
- Fruit rolls
- Lettuce wrapped around ham, cheese, turkey, or roast beef
- Rice cakes (check with the manufacturer; not all are gluten-free)
- Hard-boiled eggs or deviled eggs
- Applesauce
- Apples dipped in caramel or peanut butter (if you're sending apples in a lunchbox, remember to pour lemon juice over the slices; that will keep them from turning brown)
- Individually packaged pudding
- Jello
- Yogurt
- Fruit cups (individually packaged cups are great for lunchboxes)
- Fruit snacks (like Farley's brand)
- High-protein bars (e.g., Tiger's Milk, GeniSoy)

    ◆ Nuts

    ◆ Marshmallows

    ◆ Trail mix

       ➤ Combine peanuts, M&Ms, dried fruit, chocolate chips, and other trail mix items for a great "on-the-go" snack.

       ➤ Beware of commercial trail mixes—they often roll their date pieces in oat flour.

    ◆ The occasional candy bar or other junk food treat (see Chapter 15 for information on safe junk food)

So, Your Kid's a Little Picky…

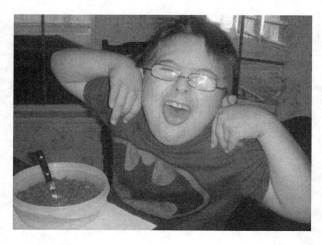

All children can be picky at times. But sometimes kids with food intolerances can be particularly finicky because they have a negative association with food—when they eat certain foods, it makes them feel icky. Some kids with autism or other developmental disabilities develop food "jags" or preferences, and it's hard to steer them away from those foods. Hang in there; here are a few ideas that may help.

◆ *Use fun and unusual eating utensils.* There are many different types of entertaining straws, plates, cups, and utensils that will pique your child's interest in food. Make sure mealtime doesn't *always* turn into playtime, however, or you'll be scraping "Rocket Raisins" off the top of the fridge for weeks.

◆ *Make the food look fun.* Whether you cut the food into interesting shapes or letters, make faces on the sandwiches, or dye the food fun colors, the way your child's food *looks* is just as important to him as how it tastes. Shaping your kids' food into letters can be a fun way to practice reading and spelling, too.

◆ *Ask your child to help plan the menu.* Sometimes we forget to ask our kids what *they* want to eat. Oh sure, giving them the freedom to select their own menus all the time may result in a diet consisting solely of pizza and peanut butter, but you might be surprised at how reasonable they can be. By sitting down together and planning an entire week's menu in advance, you will have the opportunity to discuss proper nutrition, practicality, and how to make healthy food choices. Once your child has suggested a certain food, you may find he exaggerates the meal's virtues, simply because it was his idea. Let him think whatever he wants, as long as he eats his broccoli!

◆ *Redundancy is okay.* If your child wants to eat the same dinner every day of the week, that's okay! We tend to think that variety is important, and to some extent that's true. But really, as long as his diet has a healthy balance of protein, vitamins, and other essential nutrients, it truly doesn't matter if your child eats the same thing for dinner seven nights a week. Keep in mind that this pattern probably won't go on forever. Furthermore, you should be thankful. It makes deciding what to have for dinner so easy!

◆ *K.I.S.S.: Keep It Simple, Supermom.* I know, it's not very gratifying to boil up some gluten-free pasta and drop a dollop of butter on it. We sometimes get carried away making gourmet meals that look pretty and make the kitchen smell good, but we need to remember that kids like it simple. Especially the picky ones.

◆ *Don't make a big deal of it.* As frustrating as it can be to have a picky eater, it could be that you've unknowingly entered into a battle of wills. And we *all* know who always wins those food battles between parent and child. Calmly explain that it's okay if he doesn't want to eat his dinner, but whatever you do, don't let him have a snack afterwards! He won't starve to death, and you can bet that you'll make a point that extends far beyond that meal.

14

Making Nutrition Your Mission

"I've discovered lots of gluten-free/casein-free goodies my daughter can eat, but I'd like to take a more nutritious approach. Are there nutrients she's missing on a gluten-free diet? Obviously whole grains are a no-no—how do I focus on keeping her healthy and gluten-free?"

—James L.

Know what the number-one "vegetable" in America is? The potato (technically it's a tuber)—in the form of French fries. Know what comes in a close second? Tomatoes (technically a fruit)—in the form of ketchup. Yes, ketchup and fries are gluten-free, but nutritionally speaking, they're abysmal!

You don't need to compromise on nutrition just because you're eliminating gluten and maybe casein too. In fact, a gluten-free (and casein-free) diet can be one of the healthiest approaches you can take!

Being gluten-free is a great start, but just because a food is gluten-free doesn't mean it's healthy.

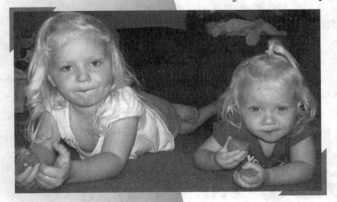

There are really three ways to "do" gluten-free:

1. super nutritious,
2. not so nutritious, and
3. somewhere in between.

Unfortunately, when embarking on the gluten-free lifestyle, people tend to end up in the "not-so-nutritious" category for a variety of reasons. For one, we often turn to starchy standbys that have little or no nutritional value. We know that rice, corn, and potatoes are gluten-free, so that's what we load up on. But for the most part, rice, corn, and potatoes are worthless, worthless, and worthless again when it comes to nutritional value.

Maybe you're thinking, "WHAT?!? I thought those were vegetables and good for us!" You're sort of right—they're natural and wholesome, and that's good. But we're taking nutrition to the next level in this chapter, and you'll see that there are healthier choices you can make.

One of the reasons we gravitate toward these foods, and especially when it comes to feeding hungry kids, is because they're starchy, fill-me-up foods. Ironically, though, starchy foods such as rice, corn, potatoes, and wheat (now off-limits, I realize) may fill you up temporarily, but they actually mess with your blood-sugar levels and make you feel hungrier than if you hadn't eaten them. I'll talk more about why that is in this chapter.

Another reason people end up taking a less-than-healthy approach to being gluten-free is because we overcompensate for what we can't have by loading up on GF goodies like cookies, brownies, cakes, and "replacement foods" (gluten-free varieties of the foods we usually eat that have gluten in them). When we're feeding our kids, the temptation to overcompensate with the GF goodies is magnified because we want them to have all the same kinds of foods that other kids eat. We get so excited when we find a treat they can eat that we tend to overdo it.

Treats are fine—and are actually an important part of raising happy, healthy, gluten-free (and casein-free) kids. But understanding and teaching your children the healthiest approach is crucial. At least then when you (and they) are making food choices, you're consciously choosing whether you want the most nutritious options or the "not so much."

Teaching your kids to choose healthier foods is a great lesson for them, and will have lifelong benefits. The foods we as a society eat today are loaded with ingredients that wreak havoc on our bodies. In the last 500 generations or so, our bodies have had to learn to adapt to foods like cereal grains (gluten), sugar, and dairy—because they've become dietary staples (but weren't always). They adapt—but not always perfectly—which is why these foods can cause disease (such as celiac disease), discomfort, and malaise. The healthiest approach to the gluten-free lifestyle (any lifestyle, for that matter!) is to eat what our bodies were designed to eat: meats, fish, seafood, fruits, nonstarchy vegetables, nuts, and berries.

Carbs: The Good, The Bad, and How to Know The Difference

There's so much confusion and misinformation about carbs, and it's no wonder! One day we read that you should completely eliminate carbs; the next day so-called experts say you should load up on them. If you think about the traditional foods you're avoiding on a gluten-free diet, they're all carbs: bread, pizza, pasta, bagels, cookies … you get the idea.

The truth is that carbs are good—if you eat the right kind. And kids especially need the quick energy that carbs provide, but making sure they eat the right kind of carbs is key.

I'm not good at waiting for the punch line, so I'll spell out the simple breakdown of good vs. bad carbs, and then I'll explain why some are better than others so you can make your own choices.

Good Carbs

Good carbs come from natural, wholesome sources; they're unprocessed, and in their natural state. In English, that means fruits and veggies. Most people believe that whole grains are considered good carbs (there's some controversy about this), but since many if not most grains are no-no's on the gluten-free diet anyway, we don't need to enter that fray. The best sources of good carbs are:

- ◆ colorful, nonstarchy fruits,
- ◆ colorful, nonstarchy vegetables,
- ◆ nuts,
- ◆ seeds,
- ◆ berries,
- ◆ beans/legumes, and
- ◆ some healthy dairy products.

Good carbs have lots of great benefits:

- ◆ **high in *fiber*:** helps you stay full longer, provides sustained energy, lowers cholesterol levels, helps to remove toxins from the body
- ◆ **low *glycemic index*:** stabilizes blood sugar levels and *insulin* production (more on this subject in this chapter!)
- ◆ **high in nutrients:** natural vitamins, minerals and *phytonutrients* promote health and help to prevent some types of chronic disease
- ◆ **low *"energy-density"*** (except nuts and seeds): provides sustained energy, promotes healthy weight loss and long-term weight maintenance
- ◆ **greater *"thermic effect"*:** naturally stimulates metabolism and promotes fat loss

Bad Carbs

Bad carbs are the kind that come from refined, processed foods. Here's where the beauty of a gluten-free diet really comes into play! Foods that we eliminate on a gluten-free diet are usually in this "bad carb" category: bread, bagels, pasta, pizza, crackers, cookies … you know the list. When you cut those foods out of your (or your child's) diet, you're cutting out the bad carbs!

The problem is we usually replace those foods with gluten-free varieties of the same product. Realize that when you do that, you're usually eating refined, processed foods that are made up of bad carbs, so even though it's gluten-free, it's not necessarily good for you.

What You Need To Know About Blood Sugar (don't skip this!)

You might be thinking, "My child isn't diabetic—why would I care about blood sugar?" Or maybe your child IS diabetic and you think you just have to control it with insulin. Whether someone is diabetic or not, the foods you eat and their impact on blood sugar is paramount to overall wellness.

Foods that have a deleterious effect on blood sugar cause us to be tired, irritable, and hungry. Does your child ever "crash and burn" after what appears to be a "sugar high?" Does she get grumpy at the same time? Could very well be because the foods she's eating are taking her on a wild ride.

It's as simple as the old saying: What goes up must come down. Your body is fueled by glucose—sugar. The sugar in your bloodstream is measured by "blood-sugar levels." Certain foods cause your blood sugar to spike. Chasing that spike in blood pressure is insulin, a hormone produced by the pancreas. Insulin's job is to get glucose into the cells where they can use it for energy. When insulin does this, it lowers your blood-sugar level, because now the sugar is in your cells instead of your bloodstream.

When you eat foods that cause your blood-sugar level to spike, your body makes a bunch of insulin in an attempt to bring the levels down. The problem is that sometimes insulin is a little too good at its job, and it lowers your blood-sugar levels very quickly. Then you feel tired, hungry, and grumpy until you eat another food that sends it soaring; you can see the roller-coaster ride this creates.

Foods That Cause Blood-Sugar Problems

Foods that cause your blood sugar to spike quickly are referred to as high-glycemic-load (GL) foods (sometimes called high glycemic index or GI, which is not as technically correct as GL).

In general, unless you're training for an intense athletic event or have a medical need to spike your blood sugar, you should avoid high GL foods. You can find lots of good lists and information about the GL of foods on the Internet, but it can also be simplified: The more highly processed a grain is (such as wheat, rice, or corn), the higher its GL will be.

This is another reason the gluten-free diet is so awesome. Those foods we have to eliminate—breads, bagels, pasta, pizza—are high-GL foods! So when you eliminate them, you're eliminating the foods that wreak havoc on your blood-sugar levels! By that same token, though, if you eat the gluten-free replacements of those foods, you're eating high-GL foods.

The glycemic effect of foods depends on several factors, including the type of starch it's in; whether the starch is cooked or raw; how much fat, fiber, and protein are present; and the acidity. For example, if you add lemon juice or vinegar to a food (those are both acidic), it will lower the GL. Fat and fiber also lower the GL of a food, which is why a candy bar, which has fat in it, has a lower glycemic index than a potato.

Speaking of potatoes, remember at the start of this chapter when I said rice, corn, and potatoes aren't such nutritional choices? This is one of the reasons why. The glycemic load of those foods is extremely high! The other reason is because they just don't offer a lot of nutritional value, making them empty calories and carbs.

Do You Need to Eliminate Sugar?

People used to think that diabetics had to avoid sugar—as in table sugar. But simple sugar (like table sugar) doesn't make your blood-glucose (sugar) level rise any faster than complex carbohydrates do. That's why knowing the GL of foods is more valuable in controlling blood-sugar levels than simply cutting down on sugar.

Stabilizing Your Blood Sugar with Protein

The best way to stabilize your blood sugar is to eat low GL foods and foods high in protein. Protein is sort of a timed-release form of energy that's sustained for longer periods of time. Eating low-GL foods and foods high in protein will cause your body to absorb sugars slowly, and create a gradual rise in sugar. Insulin can then do its job and pack the cells with glucose, causing a gradual descent in blood sugar.

Good sources of protein include:

◆ Super seeds such as quinoa and millet
◆ Lean meats
◆ Fish and seafood
◆ Tofu (soy)
◆ Dairy (low- or nonfat)
◆ Eggs
◆ Protein powders (made from egg white, whey, rice, or other protein source)

A Super Healthy Approach: Paleolithic Diet

Those cavemen were on to something! Early humans were hunter-gatherers, eating whatever they could hunt … and gather. They were eating what their bodies (and ours) were designed to eat: lean meats and fish, fresh fruits, and nonstarchy veggies, nuts, and berries. There were no crops or farm animals yet, which means no gluten and casein.

In a nutshell, their diet is: If man made it, don't eat it.

The Paleolithic approach is gluten-free/casein-free, and the foods have a low glycemic load.

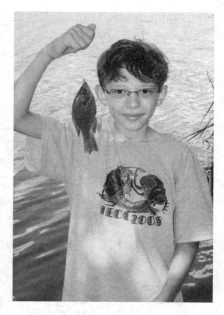

Their diet, referred to as a Paleolithic Diet, follows these basic guidelines:

- ◆ *Lean meat, fish, and seafood: Lean* meat is key in the Paleolithic diet. The animals were lean, mean, fighting machines—as were the hunters who ate them.
- ◆ *Fruits and nonstarchy vegetables:* Remember that I pointed out earlier that the veggies you choose should be colorful? That's because bright colors indicate powerful antioxidants that have tremendous health benefits.
- ◆ *Nuts and seeds:* Not only are these part of the Paleolithic diet, but they're a great source of monounsaturated fats, which tend to lower cholesterol and decrease the risk of heart disease. Nuts and seeds include almonds, cashews, macadamia nuts, pecans, pistachios, pumpkin seeds, sesame seeds, and sunflower seeds.
- ◆ *No cereal grains:* Grains weren't part of the diet until about 10,000 years ago. That's *yesterday,* evolutionarily speaking.
- ◆ *No legumes:* Off-limit legumes include all beans, peas, peanuts, and soybeans.
- ◆ *No dairy:* Want to know why cavemen didn't do dairy? What would they milk? A wild boar? Doubtful!
- ◆ *No processed foods:* Of course; cavemen didn't have them!

Dairy-free Sources of Calcium

If you're concerned about getting enough calcium on a dairy-free (casein-free) diet, you load up on fruits and veggies. Broccoli, cabbage, celery, and greens such as mustard greens, kale, and beet greens are excellent sources of calcium. So too are blackberries, clementines, oranges, strawberries, and tangerines.

Some of the healthiest foods you can eat include "alternative grains," which usually aren't grains at all (they're usually seeds). These include quinoa, millet, buckwheat, and teff.

While the Paleolithic approach is certainly nutritious and gluten-free/casein-free, it might not be exactly right for you. Maybe you're vegetarian. Maybe you want to eat legumes! Feel free to modify the approach to fit your family's needs. Again, the point of this chapter is to focus on optimal nutrition so that you can make educated food choices for you and your family.

Healthy, Stealthy, and Wise

Sometimes getting your family to eat healthier boils down to employing clever tactics that I call "Stealth Health." This is not to be confused with the age-old practice of hiding the broccoli under massive amounts of cheese and butter. That is *not* stealth health! Here are some ideas that might help you sneak some vitamins and minerals into your kid's day:

- ◆ Hide fruits and even veggies in a smoothie by cutting them into small pieces and blending them in.
- ◆ Sneak broccoli, zucchini, and other veggies into lasagna or pasta sauce.
- ◆ Use a few tablespoons (or the amount recommended on the packaging) of protein powder to pack a protein punch in a shake or smoothie.
- ◆ Buy "greens" (powder) at a health food store and stir it into apple juice or a smoothie. It's like eating lots of fruits and veggies!
- ◆ Use kefir instead of milk, yogurt, or sour cream. Smoothies are the easiest way to enjoy kefir—just mix it with berries and blend (if you want to sweeten it a little, try stevia, a natural sweetener).

Get creative! There are lots of ways to sneak the nutrients into your family's meals if you just use your imagination!

What Is Kefir?

Kefir is an ultra-nutritious fermented drink that's a lot like yogurt. It's made from milk—cow, goat, sheep, coconut, rice, or soy. It has live, active yeast cultures, making it a nutritious prebiotic and probiotic. These are foods that help the "good" bacteria in your gut multiply, chasing out the bad ones. You'll find kefir near the milk or yogurt sections of grocery stores or health food stores. Kefir is easily digested and gluten-free (but not casein-free unless it's made from coconut, rice, or soy milk). People who are lactose intolerant can usually tolerate it because the yeast and bacteria have lactase, which "eats up" the lactose that remains after it's been cultured.

GF: Healthy or Not? Let's End the Controversy!

Some people say the gluten-free diet is lacking in vitamins and fiber. The most common concerns revolve around possible deficiencies of folate or folic acid, iron, fiber, and B vitamins. But that's because some people erroneously believe that the only way to get these nutrients is to fill up on foods like breads, cookies, and cakes. Regular gluten-containing flour is enriched with vitamin B1 (thiamin), B2 (riboflavin), and B3 (niacin). Flour is enriched because when they refine the flour, they take all the good nutrients out; to make up for that, they add them back in as "enrichment." So, even if your diet is heavily laden with bread and pasta (not so good for you), you get some vitamins in there when you're eating the gluten-containing variety.

Gluten-free flours, on the other hand, aren't enriched. So if you're eating a diet comprised mostly of bread and pasta (and similar foods), you'll be missing those B-complex vitamins and iron. But this won't be a problem for your GF child as long as you ensure that she eats a healthy diet of whole foods, including meats, fruits, and vegetables. Processed foods are usually lower in the B vitamins.

Some people also claim that the gluten-free diet is short on fiber. However, this is only an issue if people eat lots of gluten-free "replacement" foods, and not the fruits and veggies I've talked about in this chapter.

Fiber is important for lots of reasons. Most people are aware of fiber's benefits to the gastrointestinal tract—you know, it helps with "regularity." Fiber has also been shown to reduce cholesterol and lower the chance of heart disease and cancer.

When people give up gluten and they load up on gluten-free flours such as rice, potato, and tapioca, they can be at risk for having too little fiber in their diets. If you eat lots of those flours, make sure you also eat plenty of fruits and veggies, or try to incorporate flax seeds or higher fiber flours such as amaranth into your cooking. Drinking lots of water is important, too.

The best way to make up for nutritional deficiencies and to ensure your child is getting sufficient vitamins and minerals is to ensure she eats a healthy diet like I've talked about in this chapter! Supplements may be a good thing too, but make sure they don't contain any gluten, and you should probably talk to your pediatrician before giving them to your child.

Your Child's Special Nutritional Needs

If your child has celiac disease or gluten intolerance and is or was quite ill as a result, she may have nutritional deficiencies that you'll need to make up for. This is because celiac disease affects the part of the intestinal tract where nutrients are absorbed. The most common nutritional deficiencies are essential fatty acids, iron, vitamins D and K, calcium, magnesium, zinc, and folic acid. As a result, your child may be lacking these important nutrients.

The good news is that because she was diagnosed as a child, she'll heal very quickly! She'll be absorbing nutrients again soon, and in most cases, her health will be fully restored in a matter of months.

As with any child, you may encounter special nutritional issues, such as a child who wants to become a vegetarian, or one who goes on food jags, or one who needs additional calories. A food jag refers to a phase when a child requests or demands a particular food or foods (generally for no specific reason) over others, then later adamantly refuses to eat this food and prefers a different food. It is also considered a food jag if a child wants to eat the same food or only a few foods, such as hot dogs, for all three meals over a period of time. Food jags are common, especially in kids who have autism. Be patient and supportive, while working to find nutritious meals they'll eat.

Lactose Intolerance

Lactose intolerance is often confused with an intolerance to casein. Lactose intolerance results when a person lacks the enzyme lactase, which breaks down the sugar lactose. Lactase is produced in the tips of the villi in the small intestine. These are the same villi that are damaged or destroyed if a child has celiac disease and is still eating gluten. This means that children with celiac disease often become lactose intolerant before their condition is diagnosed and treated. The good news is that once their villi begin to heal on the gluten-free diet, they usually start producing lactase again, and are able to break down the lactose.

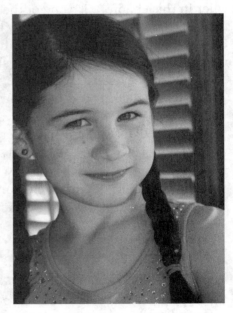

If your child has a lactose intolerance, you need to be aware that lactose may be an ingredient in other foods besides dairy products. These may include whey, curds, milk byproducts, dry milk solids, cream, and nonfat dry milk powder. Lactose may also be used as an inactive ingredient in vitamin and mineral supplements and medications.

If, however, your child actually has an intolerance to casein (a protein), then her intolerance is different, and won't necessarily be resolved on a gluten-free diet. There are tests available for both lactose and casein intolerance, but they're different tests. The one for lactose intolerance checks for a deficiency in the enzyme lactase. The one for casein intolerance is an antibody test that can be done with a stool or blood test.

Weighing in on Weight Issues

Even kids are experiencing weight issues these days. Childhood obesity is at epidemic levels in the United States and getting worse each year. This is the first generation ever in which kids are expected to have a shorter life expectancy than their parents—and weight is largely to blame. Kids' burgeoning weight is weighing heavily on the minds of parents, teachers, school administrators, health care professionals, and even lawmakers.

The gluten-free diet might be just what the doctor ordered. It's paradoxical: people who are too heavy tend to lose weight on the gluten-free diet, while people who are underweight tend to gain. I know it sounds too good to be true, but there are reasons for this.

Kids Who Start Out Underweight

Kids who have celiac disease or gluten sensitivity might actually be underweight. *You might even be tempted to skip this section, thinking weight isn't an issue for your child. Not so fast!*

It's common to see kids go from being underweight to overweight quickly once they go gluten-free. It's not that the GF diet is fattening. Done right (as discussed earlier in this chapter), it's one of the healthiest lifestyles you can have. The reason kids gain weight is because when they have celiac disease or gluten sensitivity and are still eating gluten, their small intestine is damaged and they're not absorbing nutrients properly. That means they're not absorbing calories!

Once they start to heal, they begin to absorb nutrients and calories. Kids who were used to eating lots of calories and remaining underweight usually start to pack on the pounds. If your child is severely underweight and you're not seeing the weight gain you'd like to, supplement her diet with healthy but higher fat and calorie foods such as nuts, avocados, tuna, and salmon.

For parents of kids who started off underweight, the weight gain that usually occurs once kids go gluten-free and start to heal is welcome! But keep an eye on it, because it can quickly tip the other direction and result in unhealthy weight gain.

Kids Who Start Off Overweight

Interestingly enough, the kids who start off overweight often lose on the gluten-free diet, reaching an ideal weight fairly quickly. Obviously, the delicious GF brownies, cookies, and cakes that we have available to us these days aren't going to help with weight loss. But the approach I talk about in this chapter—eating foods that are high in protein and have low glycemic loads, and filling up on fruits and veggies—will help immensely.

Keep in mind also that while weight-loss is typically associated with celiac disease and gluten sensitivity, weight *gain* may also be a symptom. So again, the "cure" is to go gluten-free and rid the body of the toxins wreaking havoc with the body's systems that sent it into a weight-gain mode.

15

Junk Food:
It's Crucial!

"I know this may not be the most important concern in the world, but are there any good junk foods that we can feed our son?"

—Brad L.

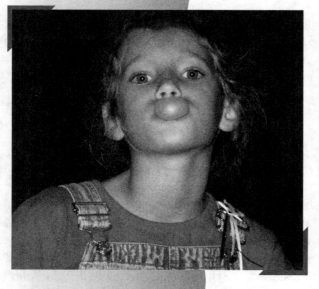

It might seem sort of contradictory to have a chapter on junk food right on the heels of the nutrition chapter. I'm passionate about optimum nutrition (and fitness!), but for better or for worse, junk food is a way of life these days, and less nutritious foods can play an important part in your child's restricted diet. Even products that are camouflaged with packaging that promotes nutritional value with terms such as "healthy," "nutritious," "high protein," and "100% fruit" are often laden with sugar (disguised as "sucrose"), preservatives, saturated fats, and chemicals galore. That's why it's called *junk*!

Of course I'm not condoning an all-chocolate-and-chips diet. It's important to ensure that our children eat adequate amounts of protein (no, not peanut butter), calcium (no, not ice cream), vitamins and minerals (no, not chewable cartoon characters), and fiber (no, not popcorn drowning in butter). (See Chapter 14 for in-depth information on nutrition.) But as a firm believer in "everything in moderation," I do think that there is a time and a place for junk food, especially when we're talking about kids.

It's **Emotionally** Healthy

For children who already have a restricted diet that can be construed as "strange," I think the commercial junk food products play a crucial role in helping them feel "normal." That candy bar or bag of chips makes a very loud, nonverbal statement on behalf of your child: "I can eat these, just like you can!" It's comforting to these kids to get a treat—but not just *any* treat—it's a commercial product that anyone can buy in any store. It's worth the sugar high you'll endure for the next two hours.

Of course, there's also the ease factor for us parents: the ability to go into a grocery store and snag a candy bar or bag of chips off the check-out stand to satisfy our kid's sudden craving or hunger pang—an act so unappreciated by most parents!

Let Go of the Guilt

I have friends who think oranges are a splurge because they're high in sugar and calories, and their version of "junk food" is dehydrated fruit with carob chips (a great treat, don't get me wrong). And I have to admit that as secure as I am about my parenting philosophies, I'm sometimes stricken by guilt and try to pretend the bag of chips I'm holding belongs to some lady in the park who was just passing by and asked me to watch them for her.

It *is* tempting to feel guilty about letting your child eat junk food, but remember the already-restricted diet he has, and let go of the guilt! You have more important things to worry about … like how you're going to explain to your zealously healthy friend how her child got a candy bar while you were taking care of him!

A Starter List

I generally do not list product names in this book. But because junk food can be crucial to the emotional well-being of your child, I have listed several products that, at the time of this publication, to the best of my knowledge, and with any other release-of-liability statements I can make, I believe to be safe for kids on GF diets. These products are not all casein free, however. Remember to check with the manufacturer to make sure the product's status is still gluten free. These days you'll be pleasantly surprised when you call manufacturers, because they're super knowledgeable about the gluten-free status of their products!

Chips, Popcorn, and Nuts

ACT II Popcorn
BAKED! CHEETOS® Crunchy Cheese Flavored Snacks
BAKED! CHEETOS® FLAMIN' HOT® Cheese Flavored Snacks
BAKED! DORITOS® Nacho Cheese Flavored Tortilla Chips
BAKED! LAY'S® Cheddar & Sour Cream Flavored Potato Crisps
BAKED! LAY'S® Original Potato Crisps
BAKED! LAY'S® Parmesan and Tuscan Herb Flavored Potato Crisps
BAKED! LAY'S® Sour Cream & Onion Artificially Flavored Potato Crisps
BAKED! LAY'S® Southwestern Ranch Flavored Potato Crisps
BAKED! RUFFLES® Cheddar & Sour Cream Flavored Potato Crisps
BAKED! RUFFLES® Original Potato Crisps
BAKED! TOSTITOS® Scoops! Tortilla Chips
BAKEN-ETS® BBQ Flavored Fried Pork Skins
BAKEN-ETS® Fried Pork Skins
BAKEN-ETS® Hot 'N Spicy Flavored Pork Skins
BAKEN-ETS® Hot 'N Spicy Flavored Fried Pork Cracklins
BAKEN-ETS® Hot Sauce Flavored Fried Pork Cracklins
CHEETOS® Crunchy Cheddar Jalapeno Cheese Flavored Snacks
CHEETOS® Crunchy Cheese Flavored Snacks
CHEETOS® Crunchy Chile Limon Flavored Snacks
CHEETOS® Crunchy Flamin' Hot Cheese Flavored Snacks
CHEETOS® Crunchy Flamin' Hot Limon Cheese Flavored Snacks
CHEETOS® Crunchy Wild Habanero Cheese Flavored Snacks
CHEETOS® Fantastix Chili Cheese Flavored Baked Corn/Potato Snacks
CHEETOS® Fantastix Flamin' Hot Flavored Baked Corn/Potato Snacks
CHEETOS® Giant Puffs Cheese Flavored Snacks
CHEETOS® Giant Puffs Flamin' Hot Cheese Flavored Snacks
CHEETOS® Jumbo Puffs Flamin' Hot Cheese Flavored Snacks
CHEETOS® Mighty Zingers Ragin' Cajun & Tangy Ranch Cheese Flavored Snacks
CHEETOS® Mighty Zingers Sharp Cheddar & Salsa Picante Cheese Flavored Snacks
CHEETOS® Natural White Cheddar Puffs Cheese Flavored Snacks
CHEETOS® Puffs Cheese Flavored Snacks
CHEETOS® Twisted Cheese Flavored Snacks
CHESTER'S® Butter Flavored Puffcorn Snacks
CHESTER'S® Cheddar Cheese Flavored Popcorn
CHESTER'S® Cheese Flavored Puffcorn Snacks
CHESTER'S® Chili Cheese Flavored Fries
CHESTER'S® FLAMIN' HOT® Flavored Fries
CHESTER'S® Flamin' Hot Flavored Puffcorn Snacks
CRACKER JACK® Original Caramel Coated Popcorn & Peanuts
DORITOS® 1st Degree Burn Blazin' Jalapeno Flavored Tortilla Chips

DORITOS® 2nd Degree Burn Fiery Buffalo Flavored Tortilla Chips
DORITOS® Black Pepper Jack Cheese Flavored Tortilla Chips
DORITOS® Blazin' Buffalo & Ranch Flavored Tortilla Chips
DORITOS® Collisions Cheesy Enchilada & Sour Cream Flavored Tortilla Chips
DORITOS® Collisions Hot Wings and Blue Cheese Flavored Tortilla Chips
DORITOS® Collisions Pizza Cravers & Ranch Flavored Tortilla Chips
DORITOS® COOL RANCH® Flavored Tortilla Chips
DORITOS® Diablo Flavored Tortilla Chips
DORITOS® Last Call Jalapeno Popper Flavored Tortilla Chips
DORITOS® Late Night All Nighter Cheeseburger Flavored Tortilla Chips
DORITOS® Reduced Fat COOL RANCH® Flavored Tortilla Chips
DORITOS® Salsa Verde Flavored Tortilla Chips
DORITOS® Smokin' Cheddar BBQ Flavored Tortilla Chips
DORITOS® Spicy Nacho Flavored Tortilla Chips
DORITOS® Tacos at Midnight Flavored Tortilla Chips
DORITOS® Toasted Corn Tortilla Chips
FRITO-LAY® Cashews
FRITO-LAY® Deluxe Mixed Nuts
FRITO-LAY® Honey Roasted Peanuts
FRITO-LAY® Hot Peanuts
FRITO-LAY® Nut & Chocolate Trail Mix
FRITO-LAY® Nut & Fruit Trail Mix
FRITO-LAY® Original Trail Mix
FRITO-LAY® Praline Pecans
FRITO-LAY® Ranch Sunflower Seeds
FRITO-LAY® Salted Peanuts
FRITO-LAY® Smoked Almonds
FRITO-LAY® Sunflower Seed Kernels
FRITO-LAY® Sunflower Seeds
FRITOS® Bean Dip
FRITOS® Chili Cheese Dip
FRITOS® FLAVOR TWISTS™ Honey BBQ Flavored Corn Chips
FRITOS® Hot Bean Dip
FRITOS® Jalapeno & Cheddar Flavored Cheese Dip
FRITOS® Lightly Salted Corn Chips
FRITOS® Mild Cheddar Flavor Cheese Dip
FRITOS® Original Corn Chips
FRITOS® SCOOPS!® Corn Chips
FRITOS® Southwest Enchilada Black Bean Flavored Dip
FRITOS® Spicy Jalapeno Flavored Corn Chips
FUNYUNS® Flamin' Hot Onion Flavored Rings
FUNYUNS® Onion Flavored Rings
JIFFY POP Popcorn

LAY'S® Balsamic Sweet Onion Flavored Potato Chips
LAY'S® Cajun Herb & Spice Flavored Potato Chips
LAY'S® Cheddar & Sour Cream Artificially Flavored Potato Chips
LAY'S® Chile Limon Potato Chips
LAY'S® Classic Potato Chips
LAY'S® Creamy Ranch Dip
LAY'S® Deli Style Original Potato Chips
LAY'S® Dill Pickle Flavored Potato Chips
LAY'S® French Onion Dip
LAY'S® French Onion Flavored Dry Dip Mix
LAY'S® Garden Tomato & Basil Flavored Potato Chips
LAY'S® Green Onion Flavored Dry Dip Mix
LAY'S® Honey BBQ Flavored Potato Chips
LAY'S® Heavenly Baked Potato Flavored Dip
LAY'S® Hot & Spicy Barbecue Flavored Potato Chips
LAY'S® Kettle Cooked Crinkle Cut BBQ Potato Chips
LAY'S® Kettle Cooked Crinkle Cut Original Potato Chips
LAY'S® Kettle Cooked Jalapeno Flavored Extra Crunchy Potato Chips
LAY'S® Kettle Cooked Original Potato Chips
LAY'S® Kettle Cooked Reduced Fat Original Flavored Potato Chips
LAY'S® Kettle Cooked Sea Salt & Cracked Pepper Flavored Potato Chips
LAY'S® Kettle Cooked Sea Salt & Vinegar Flavored Potato Chips
LAY'S® Kettle Cooked Sharp Cheddar Flavored Potato Chips
LAY'S® Kettle Cooked Sweet Chili & Sour Cream Flavored Potato Chips
LAY'S® Light Original Potato Chips
LAY'S® Lightly Salted Potato Chips
LAY'S® Limon Tangy Lime Flavored Potato Chips
LAY'S® Natural Sea Salt Thick Cut Potato Chips
LAY'S® Pepper Relish Flavored Potato Chips
LAY'S® Ranch Flavored Dry Dip Mix
LAY'S® Salt & Vinegar Artificially Flavored Potato Chips
LAY'S® Sour Cream & Onion Artificially Flavored Potato Chips
LAY'S® Southwest Cheese & Chiles Flavored Potato Chips
LAY'S® STAX® Cheddar Flavored Potato Crisps
LAY'S® STAX® Jalapeno Cheddar Flavored Potato Crisps
LAY'S® STAX® Mesquite Barbecue Flavored Potato Crisps
LAY'S® STAX® Original Flavored Potato Crisps
LAY'S® STAX® Ranch Flavored Potato Crisps
LAY'S® STAX® Salt & Vinegar Flavored Potato Crisps
LAY'S® STAX® Sour Cream & Onion Flavored Potato Crisps
LAY'S® Sweet & Spicy Buffalo Wing Flavored Potato Chips
LAY'S® Sweet Southern Heat BBQ Flavored Potato Chips
LAY'S® Tangy Carolina BBQ Flavored Potato Chips

LAY'S® Wavy Au Gratin Flavored Potato Chips
LAY'S® Wavy Hickory BBQ Flavored Potato Chips
LAY'S® Wavy Ranch Flavored Potato Chips
LAY'S® Wavy Regular Potato Chips
Maui Style Regular Potato Chips
Maui Style Salt & Vinegar Flavored Potato Chips
MISS VICKIE'S® Hand Picked Jalapeno Kettle Cooked Flavored Potato Chips
MISS VICKIE'S® Sea Salt & Cracked Pepper Flavored Potato Chips
MISS VICKIE'S® Sea Salt & Vinegar Kettle Cooked Flavored Potato Chips
MISS VICKIE'S® Simply Sea Salt Kettle Cooked Potato Chips
MISS VICKIE'S® Smokehouse BBQ Kettle Cooked Flavored Potato Chips
MUNCHOS® Regular Potato Crisps
NUT HARVEST® Natural Lightly Roasted Almonds
NUT HARVEST® Natural Nut & Fruit Mix
NUT HARVEST® Natural Sea Salted Peanuts
NUT HARVEST® Natural Sea Salted Whole Cashews
ORVILLE REDENBACKER'S Popcorn
RUFFLES® Authentic Barbecue Flavored Potato Chips
RUFFLES® Cheddar & Sour Cream Flavored Potato Chips
RUFFLES® Light Original Potato Chips
RUFFLES® Lightly Salted Potato Chips
RUFFLES® Natural Reduced Fat Regular Sea Salted Potato Chips
RUFFLES® Queso Flavored Potato Chips
RUFFLES® Reduced Fat Potato Chips
RUFFLES® Regular Potato Chips
RUFFLES® Sour Cream & Onion Flavored Potato Chips
SABRITAS® Adobadas Flavored Potato Chips
SABRITAS® Chile Piquin Flavored Potato Chips
SABRITAS® Habanero Limon Flavored Potato Chips
SABRITAS® Picante Peanuts
SABRITAS® Rancheritos Flavored Corn Chips
SABRITAS® Salt & Lime Peanuts
SABRITAS® Turbos Flamas Flavored Corn Chips
SANTITAS® White Corn Restaurant Style Tortilla Chips
SANTITAS® Yellow Corn Tortilla Chips
SMARTFOOD® Cranberry Almond Flavored Popcorn Clusters
SMARTFOOD® Peanut Butter Apple Flavored Popcorn Clusters
SMARTFOOD® Reduced Fat White Cheddar Cheese Flavored Popcorn
SMARTFOOD® White Cheddar Cheese Flavored Popcorn
SPITZ® Chili Lime Sunflower Seeds
SPITZ® Cracked Pepper Sunflower Seeds
SPITZ® Dill Pickle Sunflower Seeds
SPITZ® Salted Sunflower Seeds

SPITZ® Seasoned Pumpkin Seeds
SPITZ® Seasoned Sunflower Seeds
SPITZ® Smoky BBQ Sunflower Seeds
SPITZ® Spicy Sunflower Seeds
TOSTITOS® All Natural Hot Chunky Salsa
TOSTITOS® All Natural Medium Black Bean & Corn Salsa
TOSTITOS® All Natural Medium Chunky Salsa
TOSTITOS® All Natural Mild Chunky Salsa
TOSTITOS® All Natural Medium Picante Sauce
TOSTITOS® All Natural Mild Picante Sauce
TOSTITOS® All Natural Medium Pineapple & Peach Salsa
TOSTITOS® Bite Size Rounds Tortilla Chips
TOSTITOS® Blue Corn Restaurant Style Tortilla Chips
TOSTITOS® Creamy Salsa
TOSTITOS® Creamy Spinach Dip
TOSTITOS® Creamy Southwestern Ranch Dip
TOSTITOS® Crispy Rounds Tortilla Chips
TOSTITOS® Dipping Strips Tortilla Chips
TOSTITOS® Monterey Jack Queso
TOSTITOS® Natural Blue Corn Restaurant Style Tortilla Chips
TOSTITOS® Natural Yellow Corn Restaurant Style Tortilla Chips
TOSTITOS® Restaurant Style Salsa
TOSTITOS® Restaurant Style with a Hint of Lime Flavor Tortilla Chips
TOSTITOS® Salsa Con Queso
TOSTITOS® Salsa Verde Tortilla Chips
TOSTITOS® SCOOPS!® Tortilla Chips
TOSTITOS® Scoops Hint of Jalapeno Flavored Tortilla Chips
TOSTITOS® Smooth & Cheesy Dip
TOSTITOS® Spicy Nacho Dip
TOSTITOS® Spicy Queso Supreme
TOSTITOS® Sweet & Spicy Summer Salsa
TOSTITOS® Zesty Bean & Cheese Dip
TOSTITOS® 100% White Corn Restaurant Style Tortilla Chips
TRUE NORTH® Almond Clusters
TRUE NORTH® Almond Cranberry Vanilla Clusters
TRUE NORTH® Almond Cranberry Vanilla Clusters in White Chocolate
TRUE NORTH® Almond Pecan Cashew Clusters
TRUE NORTH® Almonds Pistachios Walnuts Pecans
TRUE NORTH® Citrus Burst Nut Clusters
TRUE NORTH® Pecan Almond Peanut Clusters

Dairy Snacks (contain casein)

Cool Whip
Del Monte Pudding cups
Frigo/Kraft/Sargento cheese sticks
General Mills Go-Gurt Yogurt
General Mills Trix Yogurt
General Mills Yoplait Delights Parfait
General Mills Yoplait Greek Yogurt
General Mills Yoplait Kid Yogurt
General Mills Yoplait Light Thick & Creamy Yogurt
General Mills Yoplait Light Yogurt
General Mills Yoplait Original Yogurt
General Mills Yoplait Thick & Creamy Yogurt
General Mills Yoplait Yogurt Fridge Pack
General Mills Yoplait Yogurt Warehouse Club Multi-Pack
General Mills Yoplus Yogurt
General Mills Yoplus Light Yogurt
Jell-O Brand pudding snacks

Fruit Snacks

Farley's Brand gummy bears
Favorite Brand gummy and fruit
Fruit By the Foot
Fruit to Go (SunRype)
General Mills Fruit-by-the-Foot
General Mills Fruit-by-the-Foot Minix
General Mills Fruit Gushers
General Mills Fruit Roll-Ups
General Mills Fruit Roll-Ups Minix
General Mills Fruit Shapes
General Mills Fruit Snacks Variety Packs
Kroger's Fruit snacks
Nabisco Fruit snacks
Sunkist Fruit Rolls
Sun-Maid Raisins
Trolli Gummi Candies—all
Welch's Fruit snacks

Other Snacks

French's Potato Sticks
General Mills Chex cereal (chocolate, cinnamon, corn, honey nut, and rice)
Hormel Pepperoni
Jell-O brand gelatin
Larabar bars
Old Wisconsin Beef sticks
Oreida French Fries
Oscar Mayer Beef Hot Dogs
Purefit bars
Zing Bars

Juice Boxes

Capri Sun
Del Monte
Hawaiian Punch
Juicy Juice—all
KoolAid—all
Libby's—all
Minute Maid—all
Mott's—all
Northland 100% Juice
Welch's juices—all

Drinks

Coke, Sprite, Minute Maid
Pepsi, Mountain Dew, Sierra Mist
7-Up, A&W Root Beer, Country Time
Big K brand soft drinks
Snapple—all
Crystal Lite
Swiss Miss hot chocolate

Frozen Novelties

Dole Fruit N Juice Bars
Edy's/Dreyers Fruit Bars
Fla-Vor-Ice
Flintstones Pushups
Good Humor Popsicles

Koolaid Freezer Pops
Minute Maid Fruit Juice Bars
Nestle's Popsicles
PhillySwirl Frozen Stix
Starburst Fruit Juice Bars

Ice Cream

(Vanilla, chocolate and chocolate chip varieties of these brands are usually GF—
check ingredients)

Baskin-Robbins
Ben & Jerry's
Blue Bell
Blue Bunny
Dairy Queen
Dreyers
Edy's Grand
Edy's Homemade
TCBY

Chocolate Candy

Baby Ruth
Butterfinger
Clark Bars
Dove
Hershey's Kisses & Hugs
Hershey's milk chocolate bars
(except crispy or cookie)
Hershey's Nuggets (except cookie)
M&M's (except crispy)
Nestle Butterfinger BBs
Nestle Chunky
Raisinets
Reese's Peanut Butter cups
Snickers
3 Musketeers
York Peppermint Patties

Chewy Candy and Gum

Airheads
Big League Chewing Gum

Bubble Yum—all
Chicklets
Dentyne Gum—all
Double Bubble—all
Flavor Rolls—all
Gold Medal Cotton Candy
Haribo Gummies
Jelly Belly jellybeans
Jolly Rancher Fruit Chews
Milk Duds
Sharie's Candies Gummies
Skittles
Starburst Fruit Chews
Tootsie Rolls—all
Trident gum—all
Trolli Gummies
Wrigley's chewing gum—all

Hard Candy and Suckers

Bit-O-Honey
Charms—all
Extreme Pops
Farley's hard candies
Haviland (Necco) Candy Stix
Jolly Rancher hard candy & lollipops
LifeSavers—all
Pez
Smarties
Spangler DumDum Pops
Spree
SweeTarts
Tootsie Pops
Topps Ring Pops
Wonka: Bottlecaps, Gobstoppers, Mix Ups, Pixy Stix,
Shocktarts, Tart 'N Tiny, Fun Dip (Lik-M-Aid), Laffy Taffy,
Nerds, Runts, Tangy Taffy, Nips

16

When You're Not There:
Sitters, School, and Other Scary Situations

"My grandson was just diagnosed with celiac disease. I
used to care for him during
the days while his mother was
at work, but now she has quit
her job and doesn't trust anyone else to feed him."

—Marion B.

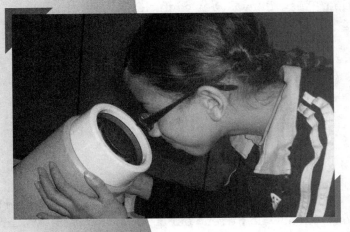

Letting G-g-g-GO!

Letting your child out of your sight may be one of the most difficult steps you take. But it's important for your child and for you. If you're well prepared, and if you prepare the people around you, you will be at ease leaving your child at school, daycare, church, camps, and in the care of babysitters, grand-parents, friends, and other caretakers.

If you have truly given your child responsibility for her diet, depending upon her age and developmental stage, she should be able to make good food choices while you're away. Stress the importance of not cheating, and then give her a chance to prove herself.

Mistakes will be made, but everyone will learn from them. Remember my mantra: *Deal with it; don't dwell on it.*

Babysitters in Your Home

Having caretakers in your home should cause little or no concern to you if you've followed some of the guidelines outlined early on in this book.

◆ *Educate the caretaker.* Make sure the person watching your child has a good grasp of the diet and its importance. Give him or her a copy of this book. Go over product information, focusing most on your child's favorite foods and likely temptations. Discuss menu and snack ideas, and provide lists of safe and forbidden ingredients. The sitter needs to know that if your child does accidentally get gluten, it's not an emergency. There is no need to panic or to call 911 or a doctor. They don't need to call you immediately, but should let you know when you get home.

◆ *Leave pre-prepared food.* It's best if you can leave an entire meal, fully prepared, so there are no questions or mistakes. If you don't have time to prepare something in advance, leave a frozen entree that you know is okay.

◆ *Remember your notebook.* Remember that notebook that I suggested putting together early in this book? The one with all of the product information, manufacturers' correspondence, and general information on your child's condition? Leave it out where the babysitter can refer to it, if necessary.

◆ *Mark foods and plastic ware.* Hopefully, you have been marking all of your containers and products, as well as your plastic ware with leftovers, with a clear "gluten-free" designation. This will avoid any confusion when your child decides that it's time for an after-dinner snack.

◆ *Show the sitter the gluten-free treats drawer.* Instruct the sitter that your child's treats may come *only* from this area. Now is when having a separate drawer or cupboard will really pay off.

School

Anyone who has walked their child to her first day of kindergarten and spent the rest of the day crying knows it's hard enough to send the kids to school when they *don't* have dietary restrictions. But how do we send our children to school—where they'll be away from us for hours, day after day, snacking, eating lunch, swapping food items with friends, and enjoying birthday parties and holiday festivities—without our supervision?

With planning and preparation, it can be done. There *will* be mistakes, so brace yourself for the frustration. With a little extra effort on your part, though, the accidents will be minimal, and you can send your child to school with peace of mind.

◆ *Educate your teachers and principal.* Set a meeting with your child's teacher(s) and principal. The best time to do this is a day or two before school starts for the year. The teachers are usually at school setting up their classrooms, but they're not yet distracted with new students, parents, and classroom responsibilities. Provide the teachers, principal, and the school nurse, if there is one, with clear, concise written materials explaining your child's condition and diet. Give them a copy of this book, if you feel it's useful. Make sure they understand the severity of accidental gluten ingestion. Ask them to contact you if there are any questions, rather than taking a chance, but make sure you don't create so much concern that they're afraid to have your child in class.

◆ *If any food is prepared by the school staff, use your judgment.* Most of the time, the people in charge of preparing food for children in a preschool or school setting are already used to dealing with lactose intolerance, peanut allergies, and other dietary restrictions. Talk to the dietitian or person in charge of food preparation. Go over the menu plans, discuss the foods your child can and can't have, and talk about the importance of using clean utensils to avoid cross-contamination. If you feel comfortable with the person's understanding and acceptance of the diet, give him or her the opportunity to accommodate your child's special diet. You always have the option of sending in your own meals if you think it's not working out.

◆ *Give the teacher a stash of gluten-free treats.* A large bag of Halloween-sized individually wrapped candies works well, and because they're individually wrapped, the teacher can keep them in a cupboard without fear of ant invasions. Let the teacher know that these treats are to be used *any* time there is a special event during which treats will be served. Make sure the treats are your child's favorite; you don't want her feeling like she's being shortchanged. If your child has a good grasp of her diet, let the teacher know that she can decide whether or not to dip into the treat stash.

◆ *Get a schedule of classmates' birthdays.* Teachers are glad to provide you with a listing of everyone's birthdays. This way you know in advance when there will be parties. You can coordinate with the other child's parent, or send your child in with her own cupcake or treat. If there's a surprise event, your child always has the stash of candy you've given the teacher.

◆ *Find out ahead of time about holiday parties.* Check the teacher's schedule to get dates for classroom parties, such as Halloween and Valentine's Day. Put the dates on your calendar as early as you can, so that you can prepare special party food to send in with your child.

◆ *It's best **not** to risk celebrating your child's birthday with gluten-free cupcakes.* It's possible that everyone in your child's class might like your homemade gluten-free cupcakes. On the other hand, there may be one kid who takes one bite and spits it across the classroom, declaring, "What IS this stuff?" You can bet your child won't forget that incident for a very long time. You might not want to risk it.

Consider bringing in ice cream bars or ice cream sundaes. Or, if you can't do frozen foods, bring cutely decorated candy bars or goodie bags filled with candy or fruit snacks (brands that everyone knows). It will bring your child immense pleasure to share treats with the class that she can eat too (and a lot of kids like that stuff better than cupcakes anyway!). Of course, you will want to be sensitive to any of your child's classmates who might have peanut or other allergies, and choose treats that everyone in the class can enjoy.

◆ *Ask for liberal restroom privileges.* Many teachers restrict the number of times children are allowed to go to the restroom, or they ask children to wait until a more appropriate, less disruptive time. Let the teacher know that your child's condition may require a hasty trip to the restroom, and that she should under no circumstances be restricted from going. You may even want to establish a little "code" between your child and her teacher, so that she can inconspicuously dismiss herself. It's a little less embarrassing than having to ask.

◆ *Have your child bring a bag lunch.* This seems so obvious, and yet I've been contacted by literally thousands of parents who agonize over how to feed their kids at school. Some, if not most, kids bring their lunch to school anyway, so it should really be a nonissue.

◆ *Try to find a way your child can buy lunch one or more days per week.* While taking a lunch does seem such a common-sense solution to the school lunch issue, it is really nice if there is any way for your child to buy lunch once a week or so. Not for your convenience, of course, but for the feeling of "fitting in" that your child will experience. While every school is different, most lunch providers are contracted by the school. Try to work through your principal to get in touch with the lunch provider and determine whether there are any meals—or even any portions of meals—that your child can eat. It can be done! When Tyler was in school, we made it a point to have him buy lunch twice a week. Yes, it took lots of extra time and planning on my part, and a lot of cooperation from the lunch provider. And no, on those two days, he couldn't eat everything they served. But even if he could eat a side dish, it was important to him, and that made it important to us as parents.

> *"Having food allergies is stupid. I hate it! I want to eat cafeteria food, off a tray, like my friends do. They say my food looks weird. I don't like to eat my food in front of them. It makes me feel shy! It bothers them to look at my food so I only eat the crunchy things."*
>
> —Brian B., age 8

◆ *Talk to the adult lunchtime supervisors.* Kids will swap food. It's an age-old tradition, and it's not likely to stop with your child. Aside from the likelihood of getting gluten, your child may end up hungry. Sometimes your child's goodies are "better" than the other child's, and it makes your child so proud that she'll gladly give them all away, to be left with nothing. So the best you 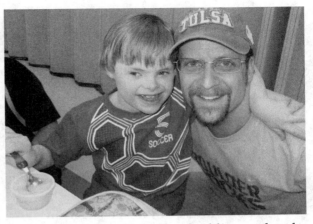 can do is explain to your child why she can't trade food with her buddies, and make sure the lunch monitors are keeping an eye out for swappers. (If your child receives special education services, food swapping is something that can be addressed in a behavior management plan, if it is a significant problem. See Chapter 24.)

◆ Learn about federal laws that may cover your child. There are several federal laws that apply to children with celiac disease at school (particularly if they are receiving special education). See Chapter 24 for information that may be relevant to your child.

Home-schooling

Some parents choose to home-school in order to avoid the perceived hassles of sending their children with celiac disease away to school. While home-schooling can be an excellent option for educating children, the decision should be made for personal and educational reasons, *not* because of a child's restricted diet. Generally, parents can overcome any obstacles they imagined would prevent their child from attending school by packing a lunch for their child or by working with the school to make sure it is safe for her to buy lunch.

Class Presentations on Your Child's Condition

Depending upon your child's age, you may want to consider giving a presentation to her class to explain her condition. This is only a good idea if your child buys into it. If she's reluctant, don't push it—you're likely to thoroughly embarrass her. Most kids beyond third grade would rather not tell "the world" about celiac disease or other conditions, but for younger kids, a class presentation, ideally given early in the school year, can accomplish many things.

Most importantly, you will be educating the child's teacher and friends. Chances are, they already realized that your child "couldn't eat some things," and they may have even been a little fearful or concerned. A class presentation will make everyone feel more comfortable, and with any luck, it will minimize the likelihood that kids will offer their food to share, or will make fun of your child.

Here are some points to emphasize:

◆ This is a very common condition, and a lot of people have it and don't even know it.
◆ Your child is perfectly healthy as long as she stays on a gluten-free diet.
◆ This is no different from kids who have an allergy to peanuts or chocolate or some other dietary restriction.
◆ It's not contagious.
◆ You might know others who have it and don't know it yet.

Not only are you filling people in on your child's condition, but you are educating 20-30 kids about celiac disease or whatever condition your child has. And additional awareness is direly needed. Hopefully, your child's classmates will go home and talk to their parents about it, and the awareness will spread.

Teasing and Bullying

Whoever said, "Sticks and stones may break my bones, but words will never hurt me" had probably forgotten what it's like to be a child. Because words *do* hurt. And sadly, kids can be terribly cruel to one another. Even comments that are meant to be "playful" or are disguised as a joke can cause heartache.

> *"Sometimes I don't even want to go to school because some of the kids make fun of me because of my diet. I know they're just being mean, and my mom says to ignore them. But it's so hard, and it hurts so much."*
>
> —Molly M., age 12

Like a divining rod seeks out water, teasers and bullies seek out people who are the least bit "different"—like your child with a special diet. Whether your child is being teased because of her diet, or because she has speech delays or behavioral issues, needs to go to the nurse's office for medication, or has some other noticeable difference, there are several things you can do.

Most importantly, talk with your child about the situation. Find out exactly what the kid or kids are saying, and address that issue specifically. Our daughter used to whine, "Tyler called me dumb." Our response was, "Are you dumb?" She'd quickly say, "No, I'm really smart!" "Okay then, why does it bother you when he calls you dumb? Would it bother you if he called you a blue bug? No, of course not—because you're NOT a blue bug."

It's a little trickier when kids are being teased about the gluten-free diet, because they *do* have a special diet. But so what? Find out exactly what the kids are saying, and coach your child with some pat answers. If kids are saying, "You eat strange foods," your child can respond, "Well, they're not strange. They may be different from foods you eat, but they're good."

Most importantly, always remind your child what makes a good friend. A good friend doesn't dump you in favor of other friends; a good friend supports you when others are making fun; and a good friend never mocks or says mean things. Pick out some of your child's friends who are true friends, and use them for examples. Make sure that your child knows how important it is to always *be* that good friend, too.

If helping your child come up with snappy comebacks and lectures on friendship doesn't work, talk with the bullying child yourself. If that doesn't work, go to the parents and teachers.

If all else fails, your child may need some formal counseling to deal with the teasing. Teasing is *not* to be brushed off as petty or unimportant. It can be devastatingly hurtful, and needs to be dealt with.

Crafts

Not only should your child not *eat* gluten, but if she is very young, it's usually a good idea for her to avoid *playing* with gluten, also. This is not because gluten can be absorbed through the skin. In fact, it cannot (see Chapter 3). But if you remember back to your early days, you know it's just about impossible to resist taste-testing the Play-Doh or the salt-and-flour dough that was molded into shapes and then hardened. Play-Doh is made with flour, and is therefore laden with gluten. Even if your child isn't a nibbler, there is the chance that some of the Play-Doh or paste will get stuck under her fingernails, and could be transferred to her mouth when she eats "real food."

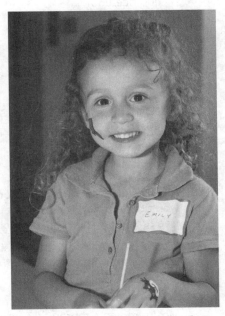

You may make gluten-free play clay, paste, papier mache pulp, and other craft products and give them to your child's teacher to keep on hand (better yet, help in the class those days!). You can come up with your own recipes, but the following recipes will get you started.

Cooking Projects

Schools often have special cooking projects. Depending upon what the class is making and how well your child's teacher understands the gluten-free diet, it may be okay to let your child cook or decorate food products.

But if the flour will be furiously flying, or if you're worried that your child may nibble along the way, there are fun options. Maybe you could have the teacher assign your child to be the class photographer during a cooking project, so that she can be involved without dealing directly with the food products.

GF Play Clay, Papier Mache, and Other Crafts

Play Clay*

1 one-pound box of baking soda
1 cup cornstarch
1¼ cups cold water

Stir together baking soda and cornstarch in saucepan. Add water and cook over medium heat until mixture reaches consistency of moist mashed potatoes (approximately 10-15 minutes). Remove and put on plate. Cover with a damp cloth. When cool enough to handle, pat until smooth.

Another Version of Play Clay

½ cup rice flour
½ cup cornstarch
½ cup salt
2 tsp cream of tartar
1 cup water
1 tsp cooking oil
food coloring

Mix ingredients together, then cook, stirring constantly, for three minutes, or until mixture forms a ball. This clay may be stored in a plastic zippered bag, and will keep for several weeks.

Papier Mache Pulp

Many papier mache recipes contain flour, glue, and resin. Your child probably won't be tempted to taste-test the pulp, but just in case, you should use a gluten-free recipe for your papier mache projects.

2 cups gluten-free flour (any mixture of flours will do)
2 tsp xanthan gum (available from any health food store)
1½ cup water
¼ cup white glue

Mix ingredients thoroughly, adding the flour, xanthan gum, and glue to the water a little at a time. Stir the mixture frequently with a wire coat hanger or whisk. The objective is to get a smooth, even mixture with no lumps or air bubbles. Tear newspaper into long, thin strips. Dip the paper into the pulp mixture above and scrape the excess off with your fingers. Layer the pulp-covered strips onto your project.

Edible Soy Nut or Peanut Butter Play Dough

2 cups peanut butter or soy nut butter
1 cup honey
2½ cups powdered milk
1 cup powdered sugar

Use a strong mixer. Store dough in the refrigerator. Discard after one week.

---

* Recipe from Arm & Hammer Baking Soda.

Paste
¾ cup gluten-free flour
½ tsp xanthan gum
2 cups cold water
2 cups boiling water
3 tbsp. sugar
1 tsp salt

Mix the flour and the cold water. Add that mixture to boiling water and allow it to return to a boil. Remove from heat and add the sugar and salt. Let the entire mix cool and thicken. Once the mixture cools, it is ready to use.

Edible Play Dough
1/3 cup margarine
½ tsp salt
1/3 cup light corn syrup
1 tsp gluten-free vanilla extract (or other flavoring)
1 lb. powdered sugar

Mix all ingredients except sugar together. Then add powdered sugar. Knead the mixture. Divide and add food coloring. Refrigerate to keep from spoiling, and discard after one week.

Another Edible Peanut Butter Play Dough
1 cup peanut butter
½ cup honey
1 – 1½ cups powdered milk

Spoon the peanut butter into a mixing bowl. Pour in the honey. Mix in 1 cup of powdered milk and blend until smooth. Add up to ½ cup more powdered milk if you want a thicker consistency. Store in refrigerator and discard after one week.

Beeswax
Beeswax has many benefits as a modeling compound:
- Beeswax is very clean; it doesn't get stuck in the carpet, in clothing, or in hair.
- Its colors stay true.
- It doesn't need special containers, and doesn't dry out.
- You don't have to make it; it is available in small sheets at teaching supply or craft stores.
- It's easy to use. Just hold it in your hands for a few minutes to warm it up and make it pliable. To save something you've made, just let it get cold. That shape can then be modified just by warming it again in your hands.

Maintain close communications with your child's teachers to determine the best way to handle the situation. Maybe you can come up with a gluten-free menu, or at the very least, ask the teacher to keep a close eye on your child.

Team Sports—Snack Time and Pizza Parties

> *"My daughter plays softball, and after each game, a snack is handed out. I've told a few of the moms about Tally's diet, but they either forget or just don't care. Every snack turns out to be something she can't eat; it's really starting to make me mad that they're so inconsiderate."*
>
> —Stacie H.

If your child participates in team sports, she will have to learn to deal with the team snack frequently handed out to each child after each game. Generally, each family will assume snack responsibility, rotating through the roster. That means a dozen or so families may be bringing snacks to the game. Don't expect them to provide gluten-free snacks for your child, and don't be offended when they bring cookies or cupcakes that your child can't have. Just make sure you have brought a snack for your child (or better yet, that she has brought her own!), and politely refuse the cupcake. If you feel it's appropriate to explain, go ahead.

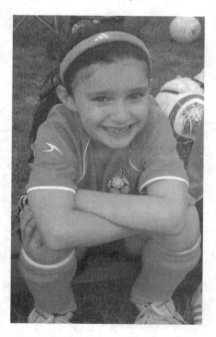

You may be pleasantly surprised to find that some parents will call you before their snack day and ask what a good gluten-free snack for the entire team might be. But don't expect that. To get agitated because other parents are not concerned about your child's diet is just going to create an additional stress in your life that you don't need—it's not anyone else's responsibility to accommodate your child's diet.

After games, especially victories, it seems everyone shouts, "Let's go out for burgers without the bun!" Well, okay, it's really pizza they're shouting for, but one can dream. So how to handle the pizza party victory celebrations? You can go to the games prepared with your child's gluten-free pizza in hand, or you can find something else on the menu that she can eat. Many pizza parlors are surrounded by other fast food joints, so you can run across the street and buy a burger without the bun, and return to the pizza parlor for a salad and victory celebration.

Religious Services and Holy Communion

If your place of worship serves cookies or other baked goods after the service, be sure to remember to bring a good gluten-free alternative for your child.

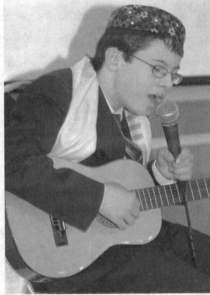

If your child attends a church in which she will be receiving communion, remember that the wafers are *not* gluten-free! Talk to your priest, minister, or pastor about how a gluten-free wafer may be hosted. Also be aware that if people have bread crumbs on their mouth when they receive the wine, there could be contamination. In the past, some priests have insisted that "the staff of life is wheat," and cannot, therefore, be substituted. But most priests are willing to work with you on a variety of gluten-free options. For instance, they might allow rice crackers or slices of toasted rice bread as substitutes for wafers.

You may want to try making your own wafers. Ask your priest if he knows about any particular requirements, and then give it a try.

Communion Substitute

6 cups gluten-free flour (or mixture)
1 cup olive oil
1 cup milk
2 eggs
Dash of xanthan gum

Mix together, knead, and roll so that it is very thin. Cut into sections.
Bake at 350 degrees for 7-8 minutes on each side. Break into small pieces when cooled. May be frozen.

You can also buy gluten-free communion wafers online and provide them to your priest or pastor to serve to your child. There are several varieties now; a quick Internet search will turn them up.

Camp-Outs and Away-Camps

Ah, s'mores by the campfire. But not for your child, right? Wrong! Most chocolate is gluten-free, and many commercial brands of marshmallows are, too. Your child *will* have to do without the graham cracker, but there are some good substitutions. Gluten-free cookies, for instance, are even *better* than graham crackers! So again, it's just a matter of being prepared and having the right attitude.

> *"My son's Cub Scout pack is going on a three-day camp-out next month, and I'm really disappointed that he'll have to miss it. How do other parents deal with sending their celiac kids away to camp?"*
>
> —Ray H.

You're not very likely to send your four-year-old away to camp, so chances are, your child is old enough to understand her diet and the importance of sticking to it. If a parent you know is going, ask him or her to help at meal times. But remember to give your child most, if not all, of the responsibility.

If it's an event that takes place annually or on a regular basis, talk to someone who has been before. If you don't know anyone who has been, speak in advance with the leaders or chaperones. Ask how meals are prepared, what the typical meals are, and whether the accommodations have a full kitchen. You may want to mention your child's special diet, and see where the leaders fall on the scale of "getting it."

Coolers are Cool—Send Food!

If you have talked with the camp counselors about the food situation and it seems there will not be a reliable source of gluten-free food available through the camp, pack a cooler with enough safe food for the entire stay. It's really not as hard as it may sound at first, especially if you also pack a suitcase full of nonperishable goods.

The suitcase of nonperishable items can contain cookies, crackers, bread, pancake mix, soups (the kind you just add water to, as well as pre-made canned soup), chili, and anything else your child will want. Most important items on the checklist: marshmallows and chocolate! Remember to mark every item with a big "GF," so there won't be any questions during your child's stay about which foods she can eat.

Pack a cooler full of eggs, cheese, fruit, milk (probably at the camp already), deli meats, Jell-O, pudding, hamburger meat, steak, chicken, or any other foods your child likes. If there are no cooking facilities (wow, they're *really* roughing it!), she can make do with the deli meats, cheeses, and pre-cooked foods. Don't forget to load the cooler with uncontaminated containers of "spreadables" such as margarine and sour cream. It's also a good idea to throw in some salad dressing, ketchup, and mustard. Many of these things come in squeeze containers that are not only handy, but highly resistant to contamination. Once at the campsite, transfer the perishables to a refrigerator, if there is one. If there isn't one available, make sure there is plenty of ice to keep the food cold.

Who will prepare the food will depend upon your child's age and abilities, the length of stay, the type of food being cooked, and your good ol' parental judgment. If your child can prepare her own food, great. That's always best, because as we've stressed throughout this book, your child needs to learn to be responsible for her own diet.

Whether or not you should pack pots and pans depends upon the length of stay and the type of food that will be prepared. Usually camping food is prepared over a roaring fire on the end of a stick. It *is* a good idea to pack aluminum foil, which can be used as a "toaster" for a slice of gluten-free bread, or even a "frying pan" for sausage or bacon. It can also be used to coat a pot or pan that has been used to cook gluten-containing foods (it must still be washed before cooking gluten-free foods, even with a protective layer of foil).

If your child will be away at camp for an extended period and you're worried that the cooking facilities will be limited or coated with gluten, have your child bring a toaster oven to camp. Really, they're not that big, and assuming there is electricity at the camp, it can save you and your child some discomfort or annoyances.

Special Summer Camps

Some of the national support groups have kids' camps every summer. These are designed specially for children with celiac disease, and therefore accommodate the gluten-free diet without any questions or mistakes. Do a quick Internet search for "gluten-free camps" to find information on organizations that sponsor special camps.

Should Your Child Wear a "Medical ID" Bracelet?

This is a personal matter that you will need to decide. There are pros and cons, but if you want my opinion (and I'm writing the book, so I get to give it!), the cons outweigh the pros.

The obvious pro is that people will know, especially in an emergency situation at a hospital or clinic, that your child must not ingest gluten. And if your child cannot communicate well due to an injury or underlying condition, emergency personnel can check the bracelet for her name, phone number, and any other identifying information engraved on the bracelet.

On the negative side, the sad reality is that most hospital personnel will not know what gluten is, much less whether or not a particular medication contains gluten. Furthermore, if it's a life-threatening or serious situation, you won't care if it does. There is even a chance that critical treatment of your child could be delayed while concerned hospital personnel try to figure out what gluten is, and whether or not it is a concern in the immediate treatment of your child.

These are the most serious concerns about this type of bracelet, but the other point to be made is one you will read throughout this book: Don't dwell on it. To wear a bracelet is a constant reminder to your child and everyone around her that she has "a condition." There is certainly no need for that, and the long-term psychological implications could be very negative.

17

Holidays, Birthdays, and Other Special Occasions

"It seems like every birthday party my son is invited to takes place at a "fun zone," and pizza seems to be the only food offered. Since he obviously can't eat the pizza or the birthday cake, I wonder if I should just keep him home."

—Loren P.

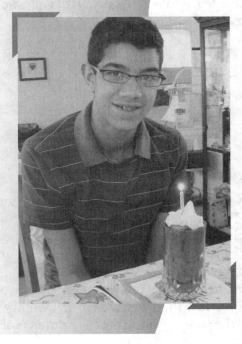

Holidays and special occasions—it seems as if they all revolve around food! These can be some of the most difficult times for our gluten-free kids. They can feel left out, deprived, and even embarrassed. But with a little effort on your part, you can ensure that your child will be included and able to enjoy special occasions and the foods that usually go with them.

Rule number one: Don't expect others to accommodate your child's special diet. If they offer and you feel it's appropriate to take them up on their offer, go for it. But to expect them not only to remember that your child has a special diet, but then to understand how to accommodate it is being a bit presumptuous on your part.

Before heading out to a celebration for a special occasion where you know food will be served, make sure your child has filled up at home. If you have a favorite fast food chain where you can rely upon getting a gluten-free meal, you could have him eat on the way.

Try to find out in advance what will be served, both for the main course and for the dessert. Exactly how you do this will depend upon how big the party is and whether it will be held at a restaurant, catered, or hosted by a friend. It will also, of course, depend upon your relationship with the host. But in any case, make sure that it doesn't sound as though you're "hinting" that you'd like the host to prepare something special for your child. In fact, you can ask about the menu more as a matter of curiosity, without ever mentioning your child's specific dietary restrictions, or else you can be ambiguous and say, "Our family has some dietary considerations; do you mind telling me what you're planning to serve so that we can prepare?" If it's a good friend, you can, of course, be upfront with your inquiries. The important thing to remember is that it's not the host's responsibility to accommodate your child's diet—it's yours.

Assuming the meal will not be gluten-free, bring a meal for your child that is as close to what they're serving as possible. For dessert, have him tell you what he'd like to have, and bring that, too. If your child will be attending the party without you, give the food to an adult in charge, and ask them to inconspicuously serve your child his special meal. Most adults are sensitive enough to be aware of the embarrassment your child could feel if they make a big deal about the different food you've provided, and will be discreet.

If you have stuffed your child before arriving at the party, or if you have provided a special meal, it's appropriate, and in fact even a good idea, to let your child take some of the food he *can* eat (assuming you know that some of the food being served is, in fact, gluten-free). However, if the plates are pre-served and there are gluten-containing portions, don't let him eat the GF items unless you're certain that they have not been contaminated by the gluten-containing foods. Even if he's just going through the motions of eating the meal, he will feel included, and it is less likely that questions will come up that might attract unwanted attention to him.

Birthdays

Happy birthday to you,
Happy birthday to you.
There's gluten in cake,
And in many ice creams, too.

The center piece of so many birthday parties seems to be gluten. As a result, what should be a joyous celebration can turn your stomach into knots.

Relax. There is no reason that your child should miss the wonder of birthday parties—whether they're his own or someone else's. A little preparation will ensure your child will have a great time, regardless of the food served.

School parties can catch you off guard, because you're focusing on homework and class activities, not other kids' birthdays. Be aware that most kids in elementary school have some sort of a celebration in school, so be sure to get a list of the birthdays of all the children in your child's class at the beginning of the school year. Mark them on your calendar right away, or you're sure to forget one, and you'll drown in guilt when your child gets home from school that day complaining that all the *other* kids got cupcakes. If one

of the children's birthdays falls on a weekend, call the parent in advance to see if they plan to do the class celebration on Friday or Monday.

Going to parties shouldn't be a problem, either, even though these days it seems that "birthday party" is synonymous with pizza. That's okay, especially if you've perfected a pizza recipe for your child, or have found a good source of mail-order pre-prepared pizza. Bring your child's pizza, as well as a GF cupcake or other special treat, and give it to the adult in charge. Make sure they understand

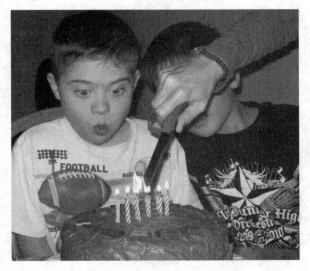

how crucial it is that your child be given his special food, and ask them to be inconspicuous about giving it to him. Remember, too, that kids are there for the celebration and the fun, *not* for the food!

If the party is being held at a restaurant, bowling alley, or "fun zone," you can still find out in advance what will be served, and you can send a similar meal for your child. If the restaurant happens to serve hamburgers, salads, or other gluten-free meals, you may be able to arrange with the host parents for your child to get one of the GF items on the menu.

If it's your own child's birthday party, plan to have hot dogs or hamburgers, or another gluten-free favorite. I don't recommend serving a GF cake, even if you make the most awesome-to-die-for-gluten-free cake in the entire universe. Chances are, there will be one kid—probably the same kid who feels obliged to tell all the other kids at school that there isn't a tooth fairy—who will decide that he doesn't like the cake, and won't exactly be diplomatic in voicing his disapproval. You definitely don't want to cause your child the embarrassment he is likely to feel when that one child makes a scene.

So you may not want to take the chance. Serve frozen ice cream bars, or arrange in advance for individual hot fudge sundaes to be made by your local ice cream or frozen yogurt shop. Better yet, put all the sundae makin's out and let the kids make their own. They'll love the change of pace!

Seasonal Holidays

Many candy manufacturers market seasonal items, and can verify that they are gluten-free. Do your homework in advance, and you will have lists of holiday candies that your child can eat. Stock up in advance, so that you're prepared to do the treat-trade when your child brings home candy that he can't eat.

Christmas

It seems like every Christmas, elves appear from nowhere, handing out candy canes like they were, well, candy! Unfortunately, most come without a label, and are therefore no-nos.

Even if you find candy canes with ingredients listed and they appear to be gluten-free, teach your child to rinse the candy cane off before eating it. Washing it makes

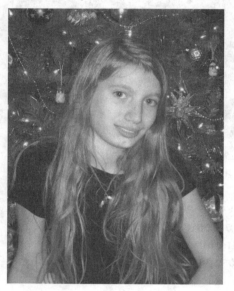

a gooey, sticky mess, but some candy canes are rolled in flour so that the plastic won't stick, and it's important to dissolve the outer layer of candy away, just in case.

There are several brands of candy canes that are verified to be gluten-free. You can stock up on them and carry a few with you, so that when a well-meaning elf slips your child a candy cane, you'll be prepared to trade treats.

Here's the really good news: Little Timmy won't have to slip his piece of fruit cake into a napkin to feed to the dog under the table . . . he can just politely decline, reminding Aunt Glenda that hers *is* the most fabulous fruit cake in the world, but he can't eat it because it's loaded with gluten.

Easter

Once again, people with the best of intentions will be handing your child goodies laden with gluten. Be prepared with a well-stocked pantry so that you can do the treat trade. For better or for worse, every grocery store is loaded with commercial-brand candies, so that you can fill those Easter baskets with all sorts of safe treats. See Chapter 15 for some safe candy varieties.

Halloween

Take the time in September to find out which popular Halloween candies are safe. Chapter 15 lists many candies that were safe when this book went to print, but remember, just because something was safe last year doesn't mean it's okay this year. If your child is old enough, make sure he knows which candies he can and can't eat, because you can bet that he'll be itching to open his treats even before he's left the doorstep and yelled the obligatory thank-you over his shoulder. Make sure younger children understand that an adult needs to check the candy before they can eat it.

Keep a treat-trade basket at home, so that your child can make an "even" trade for the candies he gets that are not gluten-free. Then do what all parents do, and deplete his stash slowly enough that he doesn't notice, but quickly enough that the fights over candy before dinner can end and familial peace be restored.

And what about the traditional Halloween caramel apples? Thankfully, many recipes for caramel coating and even the pre-packaged coatings that you can buy at the grocery store are gluten-free. But you still need to check the labels and call the

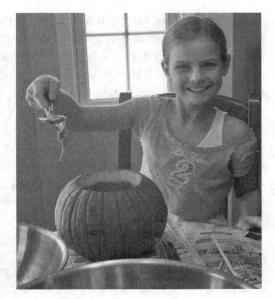

manufacturer. You may even want to volunteer to be the mom or dad who provides caramel apples for the Halloween party at school or your house of worship, so that you know for sure.

Passover

Passover is a blessed event, whether you're Jewish or not. That's because Passover is the only holiday that is celebrated almost entirely gluten-free!

Chametz (wheat, rye, barley, oats, and spelt) is forbidden during the Passover season, so foods marked "Kosher for Passover" are gluten-free, with one exception. Matzo (Matzah) is made with wheat and water, and is permitted. It is also ground into matzo flour and matzo meal, so avoid any product that contains matzo or "cake flour."

Kosher products always have very clearly marked labels, so it's easy to identify all ingredients.

Thanksgiving

Without much extra effort, Thanksgiving can be celebrated with a wonderfully gluten-free feast. But you *do* need to pay attention, especially if you're eating at someone else's home.

The stuffing, even though it is *inside* the bird, is a great big no-no. No matter how careful you are, it *will* contaminate the turkey meat. The best idea is to stuff the bird with a GF stuffing (see sidebar for suggestions on making gluten-free stuffing). If you would like to provide a traditional gluten-containing stuffing for your guests, prepare it separately and bake it in the oven. You can still pour turkey juices over it to end up with a wonderful "fresh turkey" flavor, but you won't have contaminated the entire bird.

Most gravies are prepared with flour, and are obviously off-limits to your gluten-free child. But try substituting corn starch for flour, and your gravy will be just as good—maybe even a little lighter and better—than the traditional variety. You should always assume, when eating at other people's homes or at restaurants, that the gravy is prepared with flour, and should not be eaten by your child.

Some people worry about the turkey itself. You definitely *should* check to see if the bird has been injected or basted with any sort of sauce (soy or teriyaki, for instance). Most turkeys are just fine. Some people wonder if the food the turkey has eaten could contaminate the meat. They feel that to be safe they must buy a "free range" turkey (one that was raised in a natural, organic environment, usually without severe physical constraints). While this may be a choice based on health reasons, it is not an issue for people following a strict GF diet.

Cranberries, sweet potatoes, green beans, Waldorf salad, and many of the other traditional Thanksgiving feast favorites can be made gluten-free, if they're not already. Okay, the rolls are off-limits, but are you going to be happy that the thorns have roses, or annoyed because the roses have thorns?

Gluten-Free Stuffing

◆ Key Ingredient: Creativity

One of the coolest things about stuffing is that, just as there are no two snowflakes that are identical, there are no two stuffings that are exactly the same. Even if you follow a recipe, stuffing will vary every time you make it. So, if it turns out looking a little strange, it is your prerogative to declare, "That's the way **this** type of stuffing is supposed to look."

Most kids love rice (good thing, with this diet). So to make stuffing, I start with a rice base. What goes in at that point usually depends upon the leftovers we have in the fridge—old gluten-free bread, sausage, mushrooms, and of course the "usual" stuffing elements—celery, butter, and chicken broth (GF, of course). Get creative!

Restaurants: Can We Ever Eat Out Again?

"Our family used to enjoy going out to dinner at least one night a week. Now we can't do that any more . . . or can we?"
—Susie A.

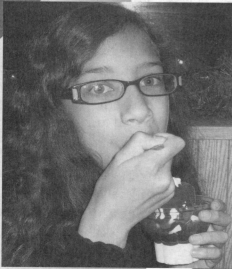

Whether you're going to a restaurant or a friend's house, eating out may not be as easy as it used to be, but it isn't impossible, either. In fact, it's much easier to go out and stay gluten-free than it is to go out and eat Kosher at a non-Kosher restaurant. Going out to eat is an important part of maintaining "normalcy" in your life. So dig out the good duds and work up an appetite, because it's time for a night out on the town!

Rule number one before going out to dinner: Always have your child fill up before you leave. Even if you are going somewhere where you expect to have gluten-free menu items, it's nice to know her belly is full of safe food.

Restaurants

If you have a favorite restaurant, you can do your homework in advance, and feel comfortable going back and ordering safe items. Many large restaurant chains have put together lists of their gluten-free menu items (bless them), and even smaller restaurants are incorporating lots of gluten-free items into their menu offerings.

Most chefs at restaurants are prepared and willing to make accommodations for special dietary considerations. It's important to give them advance notice, up to a week or two if possible, and try to talk directly with the executive chef. Ask the restaurant to fax you a menu so that you may choose a meal, and talk with the chef about how to prepare it so that it is strictly gluten-free. In some cases, dedicated utensils can be purchased and used to ensure there is no cross-contamination.

Even if you're staying at a hotel or resort for a week or more, they're usually happy to accommodate the GF diet for every meal, if you have talked with them in advance.

But what if you don't have a chance to check out the restaurant in advance? There are some important tips to keep in mind.

◆ *Ask a lot of questions*—don't be shy about it! Why is it that when the waiter or waitress comes to the table to take our order, we feel like we are allotted twenty seconds to place an order? We feel that if we ask too many questions or make too many special requests, we're just a big pain in their necks. Well, that's fine. Be a pain. Ask lots of questions, even if your waiter seems annoyed. If you get the impression that your server isn't really "getting it," ask to talk with the chef or manager. Often, if you call the restaurant before the dinner rush (before about 3:00), you can talk directly with the manager or chef. You can even figure out what to order that evening, and save the hassle of dealing with the server.

◆ *Let your child order for herself.* She needs to get in the habit of asking for the burger "without the bun," and deal with the quizzical looks. Once she is able to decide what she wants (with your guidance, of course), let her place her own order.

◆ *Don't assume.* While it's true that many corn tortilla chips are gluten-free and not fried in the same oil as flour chips, don't order nachos for your child without checking to be sure. Confirm with your server that the hamburger is 100 percent beef (no fillers added), and that the burgers are not cooked on the same surface or flipped with the same utensils as the buns. Check to make sure the fries are not coated with anything, and the oil that they're cooked in is not used for other gluten-containing items such as onion rings or "chicken fingers."

◆ *Bring your own salad dressing.* Unless your child likes straight oil and vinegar, you shouldn't take a chance on the salad dressing. Most large restaurant chains do use commercial brands, so if it's a restaurant that you go to frequently, find out what kind of ranch dressing they buy (for instance), and then check with the manufacturer to make sure it's okay.

◆ *Consider bringing your own pasta.* Most chefs are glad to cook up a pot of pasta that you provide. Be sure to explain to them that they must use clean, dedicated utensils and water. Then ask them to top it with a little butter or pasta sauce, and you have a fresh pasta dinner. Generally you will not be asked to pay an additional charge for this (but be prepared to offer a generous tip!). It's a good idea to call the restaurant in advance if you plan to bring your own pasta.

◆ *Don't be afraid to ask for your child's meal to be prepared differently.* If the chicken sounds good, but it's breaded and fried, ask to have it grilled or broiled without the breading. People make special requests all the time.

◆ *Request a server.* If you eat at the same place often, you may find that the server remembers you and your special requests. If you're lucky enough to have such an astute waiter or waitress, request him or her and ask for "the regular."

◆ *Remember to bring a dessert for your child.* Unless you check, the ice cream and typical restaurant desserts can't be trusted. Since you don't want your child to feel left out, it's best to always go there prepared. In this case, you should probably bring something small but tasty such as a gluten-free candy bar, and there is generally no need to get approval from management in advance (some restaurants do have rules against bringing in your own food, but most are understanding when they understand the circumstances).

◆ *Tip generously.* If the server, manager, or chef was accommodating, tell them you appreciate it by giving a generous tip.

◆ *Bring a "restaurant card."* You can either copy the sample in this book, come up with your own, or purchase one from a support organization. There are several

Restaurant Card

I follow a strict gluten-free diet. Gluten is in wheat (and wheat flour), oats, rye, and barley (malt). It can also be hidden in additives, seasonings, and some condiments. Please make sure my meal does not contain any of the ingredients listed above, as well as the following additives:

◆ Hydrolyzed vegetable protein (HVP) from wheat
◆ Modified wheat starch (corn, rice, or soy are fine)
◆ (Customize your card to include any other forbidden ingredients that you do not care for or do not tolerate)

It's also important that my food doesn't touch other foods with gluten during the preparation process. Please don't cook my food in the same oil or use the same utensils you used for foods with gluten in them.
THANK YOU!

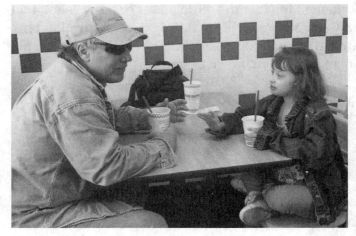

available online. The least expensive and easiest option is to make several copies; that way you won't have to ask for the card back. Present it to your server, make sure she understands it, and ask her to give it to the chef. Make sure they understand that if they have any questions, it's important that they ask you. You'll be pleasantly surprised how well received this approach generally is. Sometimes the chef will even come to your table to personally discuss the preparation methods.

Generally Safe Bets

The following menu items are usually gluten free:

- ◆ Salad. Ask for oil and vinegar, or remember to bring your own dressing, and make sure they don't put croutons on the salad; explain to them that they can't just put the croutons on the salad and then pluck them out. They can't ever go into the salad in the first place.
- ◆ Hamburger or cheeseburger, no bun. Explain to them that they can't just pick the burger out of a bun; tell them the bun must never touch the meat. Also let them know that the meat should be cooked on a separate surface from the buns, and that the utensil used to flip the bun cannot be the same as the one used to flip the burger.
- ◆ Fries. Make sure they are not coated with anything, and that the oil used is not also used to deep fry gluten-containing items such as onion rings or "chicken fingers."
- ◆ Chicken, fish, or meats grilled or broiled without the usual breading or sauce.
- ◆ Chips or nachos. Remember to check the chips and sour cream (modified wheat starch).
- ◆ Baked potato
- ◆ Rice
- ◆ Fresh fruit platter
- ◆ Eggs
- ◆ Hash browns (if made from scratch)
- ◆ Fresh cheese slices
- ◆ Cottage cheese

The Gluten-Free Restaurant Awareness Program

There's a terrific program called the Gluten-Free Restaurant Awareness Program (GFRAP) that works with restaurants to help them offer gluten-free meals. They provide restaurants with materials about gluten-free guidelines, access to dietitians with expertise on the gluten-free diet, tips about maintaining a safe kitchen, and education for staff members. You can find a participating GFRAP restaurant by going to www.glutenfreerestaurants.org.

The Atkins Diet and Other Popular Low-Carb Diets

The Atkins Diet asserts that a low-carbohydrate (*no* carbohydrates in the beginning), high-protein diet will result in weight loss. That means no bread, pasta, pizza, cookies, crackers, or other high-carbohydrate (and gluten-laden) foods.

I have my opinions about The Atkins Diet, but they're irrelevant to this book. But everyone dealing with a gluten-free diet should appreciate the road the diet has paved. Because of the huge popularity of the diet, people in restaurants are becoming accustomed to getting orders without the carbohydrates. No longer do order-takers at fast food restaurants look at you as if you're from another planet when you ask for a burger without the bun! In fact, if you look around, there are lots of people tossing their buns aside or ordering their burgers without them. We can attribute this to either a huge rash of newly diagnosed celiacs, or the Atkins Diet (and similar popular low-carbohydrate diets).

Fast Food Restaurants

You may hate the idea of fast food restaurants, and you may hate the food itself. But the truth is that they're convenient, they're everywhere (even globally), and at many of them, you can find lots of GF foods, some of which are even said to contain trace amounts of protein.

Of course, they probably don't have "burger without the bun" on their menu board, but the burger itself is likely to be 100% beef, so you can order it without the bun or even ask for a lettuce leaf to be wrapped around it in place of a bun. Some fries are coated to make them crispier, and they will not usually be gluten-free. But many of the fast food restaurants use only potatoes (and lots of salt) for their fries, and theirs are considered to be gluten-free.

Your safest bet is to contact the fast food restaurants that are closest to you, or that your child likes most. Most of the companies have representatives who will be able to provide you with a complete list of their GF menu items. If they don't have a list, ask specific questions about the beef patties, the fries, the milkshakes, and any other favorites that they serve.

You may want to ask if their fries or hash browns are deep-fried in dedicated oil. If they're not, and the fries are cooked with onion rings, turnovers, or other gluten-containing products, there is the likelihood of contamination. Whether or not the contamination from nondedicated frying oil is enough to be of concern is a personal issue, and you should use your judgment on whether or not to allow your child to eat the product.

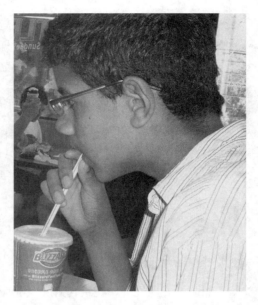

Contact Information for Some of the Larger National Chains

Arby's
800-487-2729
www.arbys.com

Boston Market
800-365-7000
www.boston-market.com

Burger King
305-378-7011
www.burgerking.com

Carl's Jr.
800-758-2275
www.carlsjr.com

Chick-fil-a
866-232-2040
www.chick-fil-a.com

Chipotle
www.chipotle.com

Dairy Queen/Orange Julius
952-830-0200
www.dairyqueen.com

El Pollo Loco
949-399-2000
www.elpolloloco.com

In-N-Out Burgers
800-786-1000

Jack-in-the-Box
800-955-5225
www.jackinthebox.com

KFC (Kentucky Fried Chicken)
800-225-5532 (U.S.)
800-268-5435, ext. 1145 (Canada)
www.kfc.com

La Salsa/Green Burrito
(Santa Barbara Restaurant Group)
www.lasalsa.com

Long John Silver's
www.longjohnsilvers.com

McDonald's
800-359-2904
www.mcdonalds.com

Popeyes Chicken and Biscuits
800-337-6739
www.popeyes.com

Subway
800-888-4848
www.subway.com

Taco Bell
800-822-6235
www.tacobell.com

Wendy's
800-82-WENDY
www.wendys.com

On the Road Again:
Traveling Gluten-Free

19

"We were supposed to go to Hawaii this July. It's hard enough dealing with the diet at home. I don't know how we'd ever handle it while traveling."
—Jim C.

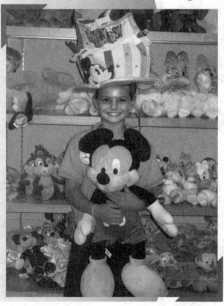

There is absolutely no reason you should eliminate travel from your plans, just because of your child's dietary restraints. In fact, it's important for your child to gain the valuable experiences that travel will provide, and it's important for him to learn to travel on his own.

How you handle your travel plans will depend upon:

1. Where you're going
   ◆ Will you be near major cities where they have grocery stores that carry items you know are gluten-free?
   ◆ Is it likely there will be a health food store nearby?
   ◆ Are you going to a foreign country where you won't have a clue what might be gluten-free, and where a language barrier might make things especially difficult?
   ◆ Are there well-known chain restaurants nearby that you can call in advance to get a list of their gluten-free menu items?

2. How long you'll be gone
   - ◆ Will it be a short enough stay that you can bring your own food?
   - ◆ Will you be gone long enough to warrant bringing your own cooking appliances and utensils?
3. Where you're staying (hotel, condominium, resort)
   - ◆ Does it have a kitchenette or even a full-sized kitchen?
   - ◆ Is it a resort with an executive chef with whom you can discuss menu options?
4. How you're traveling (cruise, driving, airlines, train)

Regardless, there are some rules "of the road" that apply to any travel plans.

Do Your Homework Before You Go

In many cases, a little homework in advance will save you headaches (and tummy aches) on the road. If you're going to be staying in one area for an extended period, you may want to go online and look for a health food store that may sell gluten-free products. Call them in advance, and find out what GF products they carry, if any. Often, if you tell them your favorite items and when you will be in town, they will order them for you. While you're looking at the area online, you can also locate national chain restaurants that serve GF items.

You might want to get in touch with one of the local branches of a national support group to ask if they know of any good stores and restaurants in the area. Many of the groups are well-networked throughout the U.S. (and in other countries where the groups exist).

If you're going to a foreign country where you know nothing about the foods, you should study up before you go. Learn how to communicate "gluten-free" and "wheat-free" in the language of the country you will be visiting. If you know someone who speaks the language, you may want them to translate your child's restaurant card into the language of the country you'll be visiting before you go. (See page 143 for a sample restaurant card.)

Learn what types of spices and ingredients are generally used in the native cooking practices. For instance, in Mexico, corn is used much more widely than flour, and rarely are processed ingredients such as modified food starch added. In Japan, the soy sauce does not contain wheat; but in China, not only does the soy sauce contain wheat, but soy sauce is found in everything. Learn what you can about native cooking techniques by studying in the library or conferring with a local cooking school or executive chef of an international-style restaurant.

Kitchen in a Suitcase

Sometimes when my family travels, we bring an entire kitchen in a suitcase: toaster oven, mixes, pre-made and pre-sliced bread, gluten-free pastas, and cereal.

If you're going to be somewhere where you won't have access to grocery stores, you can bring canned goods (stews, chili, beans, tuna, and other "main courses") and boxed items that you would normally buy in a grocery store. You might also consider mailing some items ahead, especially if you are traveling on an airline that charges a lot for checked baggage.

Most of the time, though, you're near a store and can stock up on all of your favorite snacks and meal items there. When you make your hotel reservations, you may want to specifically look for one that is near a store, if you will not have your own car or a rental car at your disposal. Don't forget to buy or bring plastic sandwich bags and small lunch bags, so that you can make a snack and take it on the run. It's also a good idea to buy aluminum foil, so that you can safely cook in ovens (don't ever set GF food directly on the oven racks) or you can line baking pans that undoubtedly have been used for gluten-containing foods in the past.

Get a Room with a Kitchen or Kitchenette

It's always less expensive to prepare your own meals than it is to eat at nearby restaurants or at the hotel. Even many hotel rooms come equipped with a small bar area that can be turned into a kitchen, if necessary.

If the kitchenette has an oven, you don't even need to bring your toaster oven from home. Use the oven instead. Just put some aluminum foil down, put the oven on broil, and you have an extra large toaster oven.

With the gluten-free items you brought from home, and after a quick trip to the local grocery store, you're set to make toast, cereal, sandwiches, hot dogs, quesadillas, pasta, salad, and microwave popcorn. If you remember to bring cookie or cake mix (don't forget the cake pan, because most kitchenettes don't have them), you can even bake special treats. Don't forget the plastic utensils and plates, bowls, and cups.

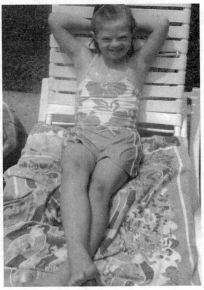

Resorts, Cruises, and Hotel Restaurants

Because they cater to people who are spending huge amounts of money on their vacations, resorts and cruises are especially amenable to serving people on special diets. Most people just don't think to ask!

Call at least one month in advance, and talk with the executive chef. Let him know your child's age, and send him your list of safe and forbidden products. Have him send you a menu that is age-appropriate, and then arrange a time to call back and discuss the menu for your entire stay. Remind him that clean, dedicated utensils must be used in food preparation, and that cross-contamination is to be avoided. You'll be pleasantly surprised at how accommodating they will be!

If you haven't called in advance, you can eat at the hotel restaurant just as you would at any other restaurant. Either bring your own pasta and ask them to cook it with clean water and utensils, or review the menu and cooking process with the chef before you arrive, and decide upon a good gluten-free option.

For more information, refer to the previous chapter on eating out at restaurants.

Airline Food

In the olden days, the best you could hope for in airline food was a sandwich that your dog wouldn't have eaten, accompanied by a wilted salad and a piece of fruitcake. Today, unless you're in first class, you'll most likely get a meal comprised of peanuts and crackers (if you're lucky). If there are meals to be purchased, chances are they won't be gluten-free. If you're flying first class, you're likely to have some gluten-free choices, but it's best to call ahead to make sure. Be sure to give the airlines a minimum of 24 hours' notice if you'd like to request a meal, and note that with budget cutbacks, many airlines may no longer be allowing requests.

As always, your safest bet is to bring a bag full of gluten-free treats that travel well, fill your child up with safe food before getting on the airplane, and check carefully before trusting that the gluten-free meal you've been given is truly gluten-free.

Hit the Road, Jack . . .

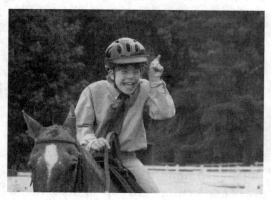

No matter where you're going or how you're getting there, you most definitely do not need to stay home because of your child's dietary limitations. In fact, you will most likely find that traveling is not that difficult at all. More importantly, it's a great experience for your child, and for the family as a whole. Think about *why* you're traveling, and focus on the joys of learning about new people, new places, new cultures, and the wonderful change of pace. Remember to keep it in perspective.

20

Cheater, Cheater, Gluten-Eater!
Intentional and Accidental Ingestion

"I thought Julie was handling the diet well. But yesterday I walked in on her when she was sneaking a Twinkie. I don't know how to handle this kind of situation!"

—Katherine I.

One of the more difficult aspects of having kids with a form of gluten sensitivity is that every time they're sick, we wonder whether it's because they've gotten gluten. We begin to question whether we inadvertently gave them something with gluten in it, and we start calling the manufacturers. Again. We wonder if maybe our kids weren't diligent in checking labels, or, worse yet, if they may have intentionally eaten something with gluten in it. And then again, we wonder whether they could be sick with something that's going around, and whether or not we should call the doctor.

What to Do When Your Child Gets Gluten

First of all, don't panic. Don't call 911 or the doctor. It is not an emergency. (If your child ingests massive amounts of gluten at one time—such as an entire pizza or loaf of Wonder Bread—

there is the possibility that her body could go into shock, in which case it would, most definitely, be an emergency.)

It's important that people, especially babysitters and teachers who may be taking care of your child when you're not around, understand that it is not like a peanut allergy or other condition in which a small portion of the "bad" food can cause an anaphylactic response. Eating gluten will not cause an acute threat to life, and does not require immediate medical attention.

Be prepared, though, because depending upon how much your child ate, how sensitive she is to gluten, and how much gluten was in the food, she *will* be uncomfortable. Usually children with celiac disease who eat gluten experience cramping, diarrhea, nausea, headache, fatigue, or some combination thereof. Some children vomit. School-aged children may have a little bit of trouble concentrating, and may do poorly on class assignments or tests. The symptoms generally appear within several hours or a day or two, and can last anywhere from a few hours to several days.

There aren't any over-the-counter medications that are very effective in treating the discomfort that celiacs feel when they eat gluten. Some people say that Pepto-Bismol™ helps; others say they get some relief from Maalox™; and still others recommend Alka Seltzer™, Immodium™, activated charcoal, or garlic. But time is the only real healer, so get used to just waiting it out.

The bottom line is that accidents will happen, and so will intentional cheating. If your child has a clear understanding of the damage gluten does, and if she gets a severe reaction to gluten, she'll be less likely to experiment.

The Five Categories of Cheaters

On a personal note, I have to say I thought Tyler would never cheat. After all, he *is* somewhat of a "poster boy" for gluten-free kids, and he's heard about the "evils" of gluten for his entire life, even proclaiming that it's "no big deal" when he was younger (see Chapter 1). The first time I found out Ty had cheated was when I ran into a good friend at the store. Tyler had been at her house for a pool party the day before, and she couldn't wait to congratulate me. "On what?" I asked. "On the fact that you found out Tyler doesn't really have celiac disease and can eat gluten," she beamed. "Huh?" I was stunned. Turns out she gave Tyler his burger without a bun, and he said, "No, it's okay—I don't have that anymore. I can have the bun." And he did.

Ty was smack-dab in the middle of puberty at the time, which is a time that many kids with celiac disease do not feel the effects of gluten (and Tyler didn't in this instance). We "discussed" the matter, since my view is that kids have hands and a mouth, and the most we can do to prevent cheating is to arm them with knowledge. We talked at length about the damage he was doing to his body, and that someday I'd like to be a grandma, and eating gluten could actually make him infertile.

He's now at that age where he's beginning to confess earlier wrongdoings, and it turns out he cheated more than that one time. And while it breaks my heart to think of the damage cheating does to his body, I do believe that he understands now how serious it is to be strict about his diet, and his cheating days are behind him.

The bottom line is that occasionally, a child will continually "make mistakes" or intentionally cheat. It's helpful to understand why a child cheats in the first place.

1. Doesn't Feel Any Symptoms

The kids who don't suffer any reaction when they eat gluten are notorious cheaters. And why not? They don't feel anything. Trying to tell them not to cheat on the GF diet is as hard as trying to convince a teenager to stay out of the sun because it will cause her to have wrinkles or skin cancer when she's forty. Yeah, so what? I'm not forty now, and I won't be for *eons*, so what's the big deal?

While most children with celiac disease or gluten sensitivities suffer greatly when even trace amounts of gluten are ingested, it is not uncommon for children with these conditions to be asymptomatic (feel no symptoms when they eat gluten) or suffer only mildly. As Chapter 21 explains, teens entering puberty often go through a "honeymoon phase" in which they feel no effects whatsoever from gluten. And if you have chosen to put your child on the GF diet for autism or other reasons, there may be no reaction whatsoever.

If your child doesn't experience the physical discomfort, you miss out on the wonderful power of aversion therapy. It's tough to break the cheating habit for kids who don't feel bad when they eat gluten, but there are some suggestions for dealing with your little cheater in the latter part of this chapter.

2. In Denial: Has Something to Prove

Anyone can go through denial, believing that the diagnosis of celiac disease (or another condition) was incorrect. People who feel no symptoms are extremely likely to experience denial, but so are people who suffer a great deal from symptoms. They may "choose" to believe that they have something other than celiac disease—something, for instance, that is out of their control or does not require a dietary change. They may believe their symptoms are attributed to irritable bowel syndrome (IBS), stress, or lactose intolerance.

In an effort (usually subconscious) to "prove" to themselves and others that they do not have celiac disease, they will intentionally eat gluten, and then usually suffer greatly for it. They may then suppress their discomfort, minimizing its severity, or they may attribute it to a different condition.

The cheater in denial who is testing herself with gluten is playing with fire, and will likely learn quickly that the one she's hurting the most is herself. With many kids, this "testing process" is just what the doctor ordered to *confirm* the diagnosis!

3. Just Doesn't Care

There are some people who just don't care. They don't care that they are doing significant damage to themselves internally. They don't care that they suffer gastro-intestinal distress. It's more important to them that they be like everyone else, or that they not be inconvenienced with the dietary restrictions of a gluten-free lifestyle.

These kids are going to cheat. The best you can do is continue to educate your child about the harm gluten is doing to her body, and hope that it's just a phase. Sometimes having a doctor discuss her condition with her is effective, since some kids are more likely to believe something if it doesn't come from their parents. Doctors hold a little more credibility than parents. (Sadly, with some kids at some ages, just about *anyone* is more credible than parents!) Even if your doctor can't convince your child of the importance of sticking to the diet, don't give up. Most kids do, eventually, learn to care.

4. Curious about Foods She's Never Tasted

It's very common for kids to be curious about what "the other kind" of food tastes like, especially if it has been a long time since they've had anything with gluten in it. These kids will sneak a little taste every now and then, but generally return to their strict adherence to a gluten-free diet, especially when they get that not-so-subtle reminder of how "the other kind" of food makes them feel.

5. Defeated

Kids and grown-ups alike fall into this category from time to time. These people feel that it's too hard to be 100 percent gluten-free. They figure if they're going to be getting a little gluten, they might as well be getting a lot, and they tend to be some of the worst cheaters of all.

5- to 12-Year-Olds: Armed and Dangerous

Kids this age tend to make a lot of mistakes in selecting "safe" foods. It's not that they're intentionally cheating. It's actually because they know too much. They know, for instance, that they can eat chips. But what they don't always know, or conveniently choose to forget (in the case of the ten- to twelve-year-olds), is that they can't eat *all* chips. The best you can do is talk to them when they make mistakes; explain how they can make a better decision in the future; and remind them that if they don't know for sure, they shouldn't eat it.

Dealing with Cheaters

Because kids have minds, hands, and mouths of their own, you're not going to be able to stop a cheater who wants to cheat. But there are some things you can do that might help.

1. Make Sure Your Child Understands the Consequences

Don't preach, don't lecture, and whatever you do, don't nag. But make sure your child has a clear understanding that even the most minute traces of gluten can cause damage. Even if it's just a tiny bite of something she's not supposed to eat—cheating can cause harm to her body.

2. Explain That 100 Percent Gluten-Free Is Unrealistic

If your child is feeling defeated by the diet, it may be that she's discouraged that every now and then she inadvertently gets some gluten, and can't seem to maintain 100 percent gluten-free status. She needs to know that's okay. No one can be 100 percent gluten-free all the time, because accidents do happen. Explain that all she can do is try her hardest to stick to the diet, and that you're proud of her high expectations and discipline.

3. Encourage Her to Ask about "Normal" Foods

A lot of kids are curious about what "normal" food tastes like, especially when they have been on a GF diet for a long time.

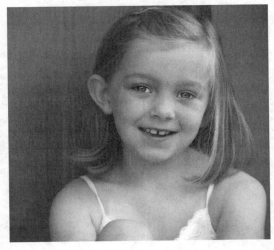

When your child asks, "What does your pizza taste like?" it might be tempting to say, "Oh, it's not as good as yours." Don't compare. First of all, your child won't believe you, and you'll lose all credibility. Secondly, most likely you'll be lying, and parents don't do that well. Rather than comparing, *tell* her what it tastes like! Try, though, to describe tastes that just happen to be in her pizza, too. Like the tomato sauce, the cheese, the pepperoni—she won't realize this at a conscious level, but subconsciously she'll be thinking, "Yeah, that's what I like about my pizza, too!"

Make sure your child feels comfortable asking about your food when she is curious. Some kids are so perceptive and sensitive to *your* feelings that they don't want to make you feel guilty, or feel sorry for them. So they just don't ask. But all kids on a restricted diet wonder about the foods they can't have, so make sure they feel as though you "can handle it."

Part of making sure your child feels that she can talk to you about her feelings requires that you be honest with her. Don't try to hide the big hot pretzel behind your back when she walks into the room. Unless your family is 100 percent gluten-free, she knows that other people eat gluten. If you hide it, and especially if you get caught hiding it, she'll feel that you're trying to spare her from feeling bad that she can't have something—and she'll draw the conclusion that she must be, in fact, missing out on something good.

4. Get Annual Blood Tests

Most doctors will tell you that children with celiac disease should have the gluten antibody blood test annually, at least for a few years, just to make sure they aren't inadvertently getting gluten in their diets. (See Chapter 22.) In many cases, the annual testing is covered by standard indemnity, HMO, and PPO health plans. While annual testing is a good idea simply from a health maintenance standpoint, it has an additional benefit if you have a cheater on your hands. If you start the annual testing early, she will come to expect the test, and she'll know that she's going to get caught if she cheats.

Don't use the blood test as a threat. If you suspect she's cheating, it might be tempting to threaten her with a blood test to see for sure. It's really better to let her know that the tests are part of an ongoing annual check-up, as recommended by your physician. Let the doctor be the fall guy!

(If you have a child with autism or another condition who doesn't have a diagnosed gluten sensitivity, you won't be getting the blood tests. Your child would never show a response, whether she is cheating or not.)

It's Never Okay to Cheat

"We're really good about sticking to the diet, and I know Derek never cheats. But he won first place in the science fair, and the judges gave out cupcakes to the top three winners to congratulate them. We thought maybe just this once it would be okay for him to have just a little. After all, we're so good most of the time."

—Natalie G.

But it's her birthday! Isn't it okay for her to have just one teeny tiny bite of "regular" cake? Nope. For one thing, any parent who has made the mistake of saying, "Okay, just this once" knows that children have a special processor in their ears that translates that to, "Okay, any time you want." Rare is the child who thinks to herself, "Gee, I'd really like to have that, but Mommy said 'just this once,' so I'm not even going to ask again." Yeah, right. It might start as a little birthday treat, and next thing you know your child will be pointing out that Fridays are special days, too.

More importantly, from a health standpoint, that teeny tiny bite of cake is poison to your child's system. And psychologically, you're sending a hugely conflicting message to your child if you allow gluten "for special treats." You've told her how bad it is for her body; to allow an indulgence for a special occasion is like saying, "It's your birthday, so I'll let you harm your body and suffer the discomfort for several days in celebration. But just this once."

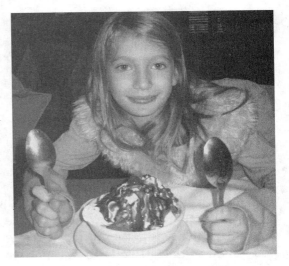

Are There Any Real "Antidotes" to Gluten?

There have been claims recently that various enzymes will assist in the "breakdown" of gluten, and may therefore be helpful to people with celiac disease who accidentally or intentionally ingest gluten.

One such product claims to contain enzymes that completely break down the proteins in grains (gluten) and dairy products (casein). The manufacturers claim that this product results in a more complete breakdown of casein and gluten molecules, minimizing the absorption of peptides and protein fragments through the intestinal lining into the bloodstream.

As tempting as it may be to use a product like this as an "antidote" to gluten, be extremely wary. Joseph A. Murray, M.D., of the Mayo Clinic, says, "There is no evidence that it will prevent the damaging effects of gluten in people with a gluten intolerance. It is unlikely that it would be so efficient as to get rid of all of the gluten that has been swallowed. I would not recommend it as a treatment for celiac disease."

Do As I Say, Not As I Do

If you're on a special diet and you cheat, should you tell your child about how you cheated and suffered the consequences in order to illustrate why she shouldn't cheat? No! For one thing, you won't possibly be able to articulate the consequences you suffered. Did you gain a few pounds when you cheated on a weight loss diet? Did you suffer a blood sugar imbalance on a diet to control diabetes? No matter what consequences you suffered, your child won't be able to empathize.

Again, kids have some special processor in their ears that translates our grown-up language into something they'd rather hear. If you say, "I cheated on my diet, and it took me months to heal," what they hear is, "I cheated on my diet, but it was no big deal." After all, what they see is the same old mom or dad. They can't tell if you gained a few pounds or felt a diabetic drop in blood sugar. In fact, to them you seem perfectly fine, so the obvious conclusion now that you've admitted you cheated is that it must not have done any harm at all!

Tattling on the Cheater

No one likes a tattletale. But I think most parents agree that when it's a matter of safety, we need to hear about it. So what should you do if your child eats gluten and a sibling tells on her?

It depends on whether the act was intentional or an accident. If it was intentional, you should let the tattletale know that it was a good thing to tell you about it, and deal with your little cheater as you feel appropriate. But if it was an accident and little sister felt a need to tattle, it probably indicates that your gluten-free child was not going to tell you on her own. That's a good chance for you to talk with her about how important it is for her to let you know when she's made a mistake, and that you aren't going to punish her. Unfortunately, she'll be dealing with punishment of her own.

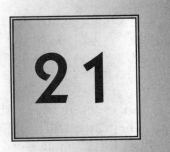

21

Celiac Teens: Not Just Gluten Intolerant, But Parent Intolerant, Too

"Kary was diagnosed at age three, and did fine with the diet—until she turned thirteen. Now it seems she's always threatening to go off the diet, using it almost as a weapon against me. It used to be so much easier. I wonder what happened."

—Larry M.

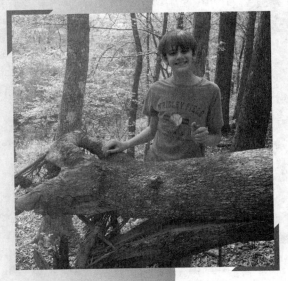

I've experienced all the ages. Tyler was barely two when he was diagnosed, and before I could blink twice, he was moving out as a young man. He has a younger sister, too—so I know teens. Fortunately, my kids' teen years were pretty easy, but easy or not, there are challenges when it comes to having teens—or *being* teens—leading a gluten-free lifestyle.

If your child was gluten-free well before adolescence, you may have just been sailing along with a child who took full control of his diet and never had the desire to cheat or tempt gluten-laden fate. Then adolescence hits, and suddenly he's heading for the pizza parlor for "the real thing" and telling you there's nothing you can do about it.

As though the challenges of dealing with teenagers weren't enough, dealing with teenagers who have dietary restrictions can be—well, let's just say "difficult" and leave it at that.

Perhaps some of you are thinking, "*My* teenager is a dream and isn't going through that typical teen rebellion that my friends talk about." Well, then you can skip this chapter—or maybe you'll want to read it for your "friends" who have typical teens. And then again, you could wait five minutes for your teen's next mood to hit.

The bottom line is that teens act differently because they *are* different. They experience immense physical, intellectual, and emotional changes, all in a very short period of time. During this time they have amazing powers. They can transform themselves from Beaver Cleaver into Freddy Krueger in a matter of five minutes or less. They can turn a glorious family reunion into a scene from *The Exorcist* with one wrong word. They can interpret "Please clean up your room" as "I hate you, love your brother more, and wish you had never been born." Their emotional roller coasters would be the envy of any amusement park designer.

One of the most significant of all emotional changes is that they feel a sense of independence, power, and control over their bodies and their lives that they cannot ignore. Their lives transform from being dominated by their parents to being dominated by themselves. They forcefully and purposefully *push* their childhood behind—and pull away from their parents' grasp.

Letting G-g-g-g-go

Just as it's their job to grow up, it's *your* job to let go. I'm not sure if it's more difficult to let go because you're afraid they still need you, or because you're afraid they won't.

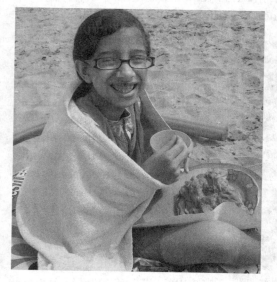

The hardest part of letting go at this point is that you can't let go completely. You have to find and then walk that fine line of letting go enough that they learn to conquer the world on their own, yet still maintain enough control that you are setting limits and confronting them with their undesirable behavior.

What this means to the parents of teens on a gluten-free diet is that there *will* be times when they make "mistakes." And many times they *will* be intentional.

So, how do you respond to your child's blatant disregard for his body? You express your concern, and then you bite your tongue. He'll be expecting a lecture, so whatever you do, don't give him one. The beauty of celiac disease is that *he's* the one who will suffer most. And for a teenager, I can't think of a worse punishment than to be slammed with a bad case of odiferous flatulence accompanied by a good old dose of diarrhea.

Acceptance = Happiness

To a teen, happiness comes from being accepted by your friends. So it is no wonder that gluten-free teens have a difficult time dealing with their very special diet. After all, at a point in their lives when they judge one another on the most trivial discrepancies from the norm, it's just not cool to be eating pizza made on a corn tortilla.

How their friends respond to their diet can either make it incredibly easy for them to deal with, or incredibly difficult. While most of us assume that peers would make this period difficult on a child with a gluten-free lifestyle, sometimes we're pleasantly surprised by kids' support of one another, especially as teens.

The Teen Who Is Newly Diagnosed

Imagine—your teen's body has changed to the point that he truly does not recognize himself anymore. He wants to be grown up, but he wants to be taken care of. He has school, friends, and responsibilities to juggle, and parents who won't get off his back. The one thing he has full control over is his body. And then that's taken away, because he's being told he can't eat *anything* he and his friends used to eat.

Because of all the inherent stress factors in being a teenager, having to go gluten-free at this point could just be too much for him to handle on his own. If your teen seems to be having a difficult time accepting the condition, seek counseling immediately, preferably from a professional who understands both teens and dietary restrictions (e.g., diabetes and/or celiac disease). Most pediatricians will be able to refer you to a knowledgeable mental health professional.

Sometimes it helps for teens to talk to teens. The gluten-free community is very supportive, and if you ask, there will be teens who will contact yours and let him know he's not alone. There are even teen websites and online groups. Do a Google search of "teen gluten-free" and you'll turn up several options. Support groups may also be helpful. Contact your local chapter of a national gluten-free support organization. If you don't have the number of a local chapter, call or email a national organization and see what they can do to help.

Teenaged Manipulation, Gluten-Free Style

Picture yourself in the following situation: Missy (oops, it's Melissa now) wants to go to Tara's house on a weeknight.

"Mom, can I go to Tara's house to listen to CDs tonight?"

"No, Missy, uh, Melissa. It's a Tuesday night, and you know we don't allow you to go out on a school night."

"But Mom, *everyone else* gets to go out on a school night!"

"I said no. We have rules in this house, and that's one of them."

"But (tears beginning to flow on command) Tara is the only one who understands about me having to be gluten-free. She's the only one who doesn't make fun of me. Just today, Karen and Joanne were calling me a freak because I eat such stupid stuff. They said my muffin looked like a pile of sawdust glued together. No one else understands! *You* don't understand! Tara is the only one who understands. *She* makes me feel okay about it, and I could sure use *her* support right now. . . ."

Bullseye. Right smack dab in the middle of your heart. Button numero-uno, she pulls the sympathy card.

The best way to avoid being vulnerable to the manipulation game is to be prepared for the attack. Remember the *real* point of the conversation, and stick to your rules. Obviously, her condition and Tara's sympathetic nature have nothing to do with whether or not you allow your kids to go out on a school night. So, as much as your child tries to derail you by honing in on your own feelings of guilt or sympathy, be resolute in your stand, and put the discussion back on track.

National Support Organizations

Contact information for some of the many national organizations that can provide support and information about the gluten-free lifestyle:

Celiac Disease Foundation
818-990-2354
cdf@celiac.org
www.celiac.org

Celiac Sprue Association
877-CSA-4CSA
celiacs@csaceliacs.org
www.csaceliacs.org

Food Allergy & Anaphylaxis Network
800-929-4040
faan@foodallergy.org
www.foodallergy.org

Gluten Intolerance Group of North America
253-833-6655
info@gluten.net
www.gluten.net

Dating and Parties

As though a first date isn't stressful enough, teens who are on a strict gluten-free diet may have reason to be especially nervous. If the date will be at a restaurant, should they mention their condition to their date? What about when it comes time to have dinner with the boyfriend's or girlfriend's parents?

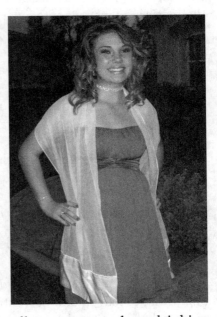

There are no right and wrong ways for parents to help their teens with these kinds of feelings. As a parent, however, you should be aware that dating may be more anxiety-provoking for your child, and you should make it clear that you are always available to discuss these things with him. Hopefully, you've been talking with your child all along about how real friends treat their friends (see Chapter 8). This may be a good time to remind him that someone who is worth knowing will not judge him by his diet.

While you're having "the talk," don't forget to talk to your teen about drinking alcohol. Regardless of your personal views on underage drinking, you and your child should both know and discuss the fact that beer and some other alcoholic beverages are loaded with gluten.

Hormones and the "Honeymoon Period"

Celiac disease does a strange thing during adolescence. It actually appears to "go away." In fact, celiac disease never "goes away," and people do not outgrow it. But usually around the onset of puberty, most likely due to the many hormonal changes, celiacs who eat gluten no longer feel the effects—at least not as much as they once did. Specialists refer to this as the "honeymoon phase."

> *"Sophie was showing signs of celiac disease for a few years, but when she turned twelve, they seemed to go away. We just figured she outgrew it."*
>
> —Sheldon T.

This is a very dangerous phase. Without the diarrhea and cramping, teens figure it must be okay to eat gluten, and they go crazy making up for lost gluten-eating time! But the gluten molecules are still doing harm to the small intestine, laying the groundwork for severe consequences down the road.

Denial—among kids, of course, but also among parents—is very common during the honeymoon phase. Eager to believe that their kids don't have celiac disease, parents begin to suspect a misdiagnosis. After all, look at them now! They can eat *anything*, and they feel just fine! It's a false and dangerous sense of security. If you truly suspect a misdiagnosis, you may want to have the antibody screening (blood test) done. But remember, to obtain accurate antibody results, your child must be eating a gluten-containing diet for at least a few weeks. (See Chapter 22 for more information on testing.)

For people with celiac disease, the honeymoon period generally ends in the late teenage years or early twenties. At that point, if the child has been gluten-free, there will be little or no change in his condition. He's gluten-free, and except for the difficulties experienced as a result of raging hormones, he should be a healthy, normal teen (is that an oxymoron?).

But if he has been eating gluten with no apparent symptoms, thanks to the honeymoon period, he may begin to experience the discomfort that most people with celiac disease or gluten sensitivity feel when they eat gluten.

You might think that many diagnoses are made during young adulthood as teens are coming off their honeymoon period. Surprisingly, while there are more diagnoses made in the early twenties than, say, the mid-teens, it is not as commonly diagnosed at this time as one might think.

There are a few reasons for this paradox. One is that at this age, young adults are beginning to leave home to venture out on their own. They may be distracted by the many other exciting things going on in their lives, such as finding an apartment, beginning a career, and becoming involved in serious relationships. They may not even notice their discomfort.

Or, they may feel the symptoms of celiac disease, but chalk them up to the new stresses they are facing. Beginning a life on their own, they may also be hesitant to seek medical help because of the costs involved.

For whatever reason, many people who begin to feel symptoms after breaking out of the honeymoon phase ignore them, and even become used to them. These people often blame their discomfort on a presumed lactose intolerance, stress, irritable bowel syndrome, or some other ambiguous condition. They will usually suffer for years before seeking medical advice, and will be diagnosed later in life—if at all.

22

A Closer Look at Celiac Disease

If your child has been diagnosed with CD or you suspect she may have the disorder, this chapter is for you. Here is where you will find the information on causes and diagnosis.

Celiac disease is the most common genetic disease of mankind. Chances are very good that you know several people who have it—but just don't know it yet. If your child has been diagnosed with celiac disease or you suspect she may have it, you'll want to tune into this chapter. It's important for you and your family to understand the condition in detail. Even if you don't have a child with celiac disease, you should read more about the condition so you understand the symptoms and testing. You might be able to change someone's life by guiding them toward a diagnosis.

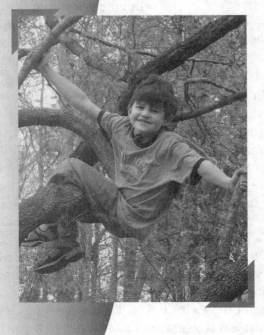

What Is Celiac Disease?

It's the most common genetic disease of mankind, occurring in about 1 percent of the population, yet most people who have it don't know it. And, people who go undiagnosed are at risk for developing a myriad of other conditions.

Celiac disease is a genetic disorder in which gluten intolerance leads to damage to the lining of the small intestine. In other words, people with celiac disease have a sensitivity to *gluten*—a protein found in wheat, rye, oats, and barley (as well as malt, which is made from barley).

In people with celiac disease, gluten damages the *villi* in the small intestine. Villi are the small hair-like projections that are responsible for absorbing nutrients from digested food (see illustration below). Eventually, the villi may become partially or even completely flattened, and unable to do their job. When this happens, the body is deprived of basic nutrients, and the person may become malnourished and dehydrated. There *is* good news, however. The damage is completely reversible if gluten is removed from the diet.

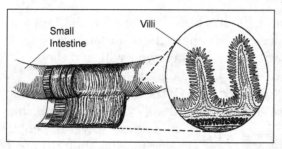

Healthy villi on the lining of the small intestine help absorb nutrients.

People often ask what causes celiac disease. Nothing causes it, although something *may* trigger it. People with celiac disease have a "genetic predisposition" for developing celiac disease. That is, they carry a gene or genes that *may* result in celiac disease under some circumstances, but not others.

Celiac disease is *multigenetic*. This means that it's more complex than being simply a dominant trait, passed on by one parent or a recessive trait, passed on by both parents. There are several genes involved, each of which may have different strengths of expression.

The important thing to note is that if your child has celiac disease, it's because the disorder runs in one or both sides of the family. Often after a child is diagnosed, parents will realize that, interestingly, Grandma had lymphoma (cancer), or Grandpa never did eat bread because he said it made him feel bad, Dad feels lousy after drinking a beer, or someone in the family was told at some point that he or she had a wheat "allergy." It is likely that many of the family members have had celiac disease, but were never diagnosed.

Genetics don't tell the whole story, though. We know this because identical twins, genetically the same in every way, do not always both get celiac disease. In fact, in "only" 70-75 percent of identical twin sets do both twins have celiac disease; in the other 25-30 percent, only one of the twins has it. The nongenetic factors are not yet known, but certain viruses or stress triggers are suspected.

What Are the Symptoms of Celiac Disease?

The symptoms of celiac disease result from the inability of the small intestine to absorb nutrients from food as it is digested. These symptoms may appear as soon as your child begins to eat gluten—usually just before her first birthday—or they may not show up until later. Interestingly, the two most common age ranges for exhibiting celiac symptoms are the toddler years (ages 1 to 4) and the 50s. (See below for information on possible triggers of celiac disease.)

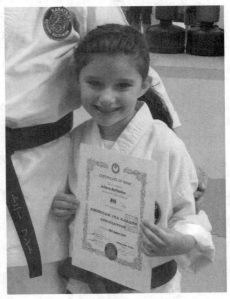

Celiac disease is difficult to diagnose because the symptoms are so varied. Some people exhibit "classic" symptoms such as diarrhea, malabsorption, gas, and bloating. Others may experience fatigue, anemia, irritability, vomiting, short stature, or difficulty concentrating.

It is extremely important to note that some people with celiac disease show absolutely no symptoms whatsoever. These are called "asymptomatic" or "silent" celiacs, but the damage is still being done! It is also important to realize that just because your child does *not* show these "classic" symptoms does *not* mean she does not have celiac disease. Celiac disease is a diagnosis based on the abnormality in the intestines, not the symptoms.

"Classic" and Common Symptoms for Infants and Toddlers

- ◆ Diarrhea—oftentimes the diarrhea is described by parents as being particularly foul smelling and foamy in appearance
- ◆ Failure to thrive (below average weight gain or increase in height)
- ◆ Projectile vomiting
- ◆ Distended abdomen
- ◆ Lack of muscle definition (throughout the body)
- ◆ Irritability
- ◆ Listlessness
- ◆ Lack of desire to eat
- ◆ Low levels of calcium, vitamin B-12, and folic acid
- ◆ Extreme separation anxiety or excessive dependence on parents (probably because they're in pain and get comfort from parents)

"Classic" and Common Symptoms for Children and Adults

- ◆ Gastrointestinal distress (cramping, bloating, gas)
- ◆ Diarrhea
- ◆ Constipation
- ◆ Steatorrhea (foul, frothy, sometimes floating stools)
- ◆ Anemia and/or nutritional deficiencies
- ◆ Lack of muscle definition
- ◆ Delayed onset of puberty
- ◆ Weight loss
- ◆ Lack of desire to eat
- ◆ Emotional disturbances including irritability, depression, difficulty concentrating, and excessive dependence
- ◆ Dental disorders (ridges and changes in pigmentation in secondary teeth)

If left untreated, celiac disease can cause a number of long-term and even life-threatening conditions, including:

- ◆ Osteoporosis and other bone disease, such as osteomalacia, osteopenia, and rickets
- ◆ Bone "pain"
- ◆ Weight loss
- ◆ Epilepsy
- ◆ Internal hemorrhaging
- ◆ Central and peripheral nervous system disorders
- ◆ Pancreatic disease or disorders
- ◆ Intestinal lymphoma (cancer)
- ◆ Anemia
- ◆ Chronic diarrhea
- ◆ Lactose intolerance
- ◆ Lack of dental enamel formation (in children)
- ◆ Infertility (in both men and women)
- ◆ In women, miscarriage, delayed start of menstruation, premature menopause
- ◆ A variety of emotional or behavioral disturbances, including anxiety, depression, chronic fatigue, irritability, an inability to concentrate, and even schizophrenic behavior.

Symptoms aside, you can also expect a little (or a lot of) resistance from your child regarding the new diet. That's okay; it's a new concept for everyone. You will most likely be feeling a myriad of emotions yourself, which will be reflected in your child's moods and behavior. Time will heal that, too.

What Triggers Celiac Disease?

Since celiac disease is a genetic disorder, the tendency to acquire celiac disease is present at birth. It is not yet understood why people get the damage (disease) at any particular age. Perhaps an infection causes initial damage to the intestine, allowing the immune system to recognize portions of the gluten molecule as "foreign." This may set the disease process going.

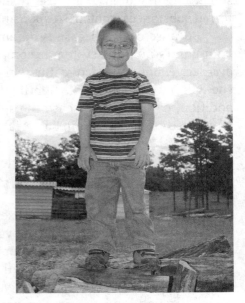

Some children exhibit severe symptoms soon after gluten is introduced into their diet. Others show mild symptoms in early childhood, but the symptoms seem to mysteriously disappear between the ages of six (or so) until after puberty. This is referred to as a "honeymoon period," and no one is quite sure why this occurs. Tolerance to gluten, or lack of symptoms in adolescence, is very common.

Yet others show absolutely no symptoms until their twenties, thirties, forties, or later. It is thought that a trigger of some sort eventually prompts an individual to get the disease. Then there may be another trigger that results in the actual symptoms of the disease. Triggers can include a virus, pregnancy, surgery or other physical trauma to the body, or stress. Sometimes there just isn't an explanation for what triggered the symptoms to appear—they're just there. And, probably most commonly, the symptoms were there all along, but they were ignored, masked, or misdiagnosed as irritable bowel syndrome, lactose intolerance, gas, or other benign and common conditions. Often people get used to "feeling lousy," chronic fatigue, or a variety of gastrointestinal discomforts.

What Happens Once Celiac Disease Is Triggered?

Celiac disease is an *autoimmune disorder*. An autoimmune disorder is a general term for disorders in which the body produces immune reactions against itself, resulting in tissue injury. The immune system is a complicated network of cells and cell components (called *molecules*) that normally work to defend the body and eliminate infections caused by bacteria, viruses, and other invading microbes. When someone has an autoimmune disease, the immune system mistakenly attacks itself, targeting the cells, tissues, and organs of that person's own body.

Most immune system cells are white blood cells, of which there are many types. Lymphocytes are one type of white blood cell, and two major classes of lymphocytes are *T-cells* and *B-cells*. T-cells are critical immune system cells that help to destroy infected cells and coordinate the overall immune response. B-cells are best known for making antibodies.

In people with celiac disease, T-cells in the intestines respond specifically to something in gluten. It is these T-cells, which usually fight cold viruses and other external substances, that are responsible for the damage to the villi.

Because celiac disease is an autoimmune disorder, you may be concerned that your child's immune system is compromised. In fact, your child's immune system is *over*active, not underactive. But while your child is chronically ill from celiac disease, she will have more trouble fighting infections. This may be due to poor nutrition. In addition, early in the disease the spleen does not function well. This makes people more susceptible to certain bacterial infections.

Is Celiac Disease an Allergy? NO!

Many people refer to celiac disease as an allergy. It's *not* an allergy, but an autoimmune disorder, as explained above.

I believe it's dangerous for people to think that celiac disease is an allergy. Some parents, believing it is an allergy, will feed their children gluten, followed by an antihistamine to "counteract the allergic reaction." Others believe that allergies can be "overcome" through a desensitization process of gradually introducing the allergen back into the diet. If, however, someone slowly introduces gluten into the diet of child with celiac disease, it is like feeding her poison. Slowly. And finally, people *can* outgrow an

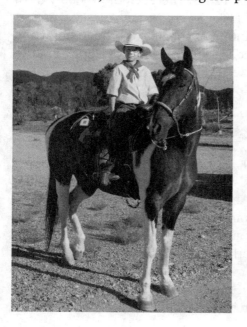

allergy. But no matter how hard you wish, your child will not outgrow celiac disease.

If you are interested in the physiological difference between an allergy and an autoimmune disorder, read on. The rest of you can skip ahead! Technically, the difference is this: with an allergy, an allergen (the substance you're allergic to) is detected by the B-cells in your blood. The B-cells see that allergen as an enemy, and produce an antibody that is very specifically designed to fight that allergen. In the case of allergies, the antibody produced is called IgE (immunoglobulin E). Histamine is then released. Histamine is the chemical that causes us to feel so bad when we have an allergic reaction. The reaction generally occurs quite quickly.

Celiac disease, on the other hand, is an *intolerance*. There is no release of IgE (it's actually an IgA response), and the reaction occurs much more slowly, so symptoms can be delayed by as much as a day or two (which is why it can be difficult to pinpoint the food someone can't tolerate). Another difference is that the effects of gluten on someone with celiac disease are cumulative, causing more and more damage to the villi every time it is ingested.

Could Other Family Members Have It?

Absolutely. Celiac disease is a genetic condition, which means someone in your child's biological ancestry passed it down. It also means that relatives may have it—and they may not even know it. The more closely related someone is to your child with celiac disease, the more likely it is that they have it or will develop symptoms. There is an estimated 10 to 30 percent incidence in first-degree (direct) relatives (meaning parents, children, and siblings).[*] Many (estimates range from 10 to 50 percent) first-degree relatives have asymptomatic celiac disease, which means they show no symptoms.[**] It is important to remember, however, that while people have varying degrees of *symptoms*, there is no such thing as having a "milder" case of celiac disease (see below). Either you have it or you don't.

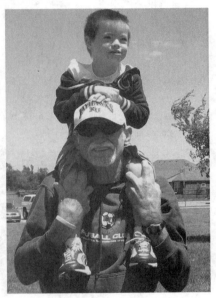

Could My Child Just Have "a Touch" of Celiac Disease?

There is no such thing as having "a touch of celiac disease." Some people may have "milder" symptoms, or even no symptoms at all, but the damage is still being done internally. The reason some people show fewer or no symptoms ("asymptomatic" or "compensated-latent disease") is because:

1. the length of the small bowel that has been damaged is shorter, or
2. there is less damage to the mucous membrane, or the lining, of the small intestine, or
3. they're in the "honeymoon period" described earlier in this chapter and also in Chapter 21.

---

[*] "Familial Incidence of Celiac Disease," presented aboard *Celiac Experience III,* January 1994 by Joseph A. Murray, M.D.

[**] Karoly Horvath, M.D., as written in *Gluten-Free Living Magazine,* January/February 1999.

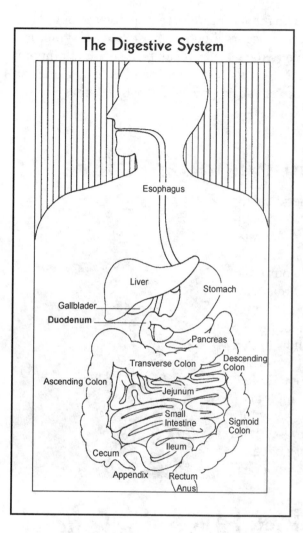

The Digestive System

Esophagus

Liver

Stomach

Gallbladder

Duodenum

Pancreas

Transverse Colon

Descending Colon

Ascending Colon

Jejunum

Small Intestine

Sigmoid Colon

Ileum

Cecum

Appendix

Rectum

Anus

The damage in celiac disease starts in the duodenum, the area of the small intestine that connects with the stomach.

In celiac disease, the damage starts in the small intestine just beyond the stomach, and works its way down (see illustration below). If the damage is only near the stomach, there are several feet of small intestine left to compensate for the damaged portion that does not absorb food and nutrients. That remaining portion can absorb enough of the food and liquid that the person may not ever have diarrhea and other classic symptoms. It's important to note, however, that even though there are no classic symptoms, gluten is always damaging to people with celiac disease. No matter how slight the damage may be, it can—and generally will (if the child isn't put on a gluten-free diet right away)—spread. In addition, because the upper part of the intestine is where iron, folic acid, calcium, and fat soluble vitamins (K, A, D, E) are absorbed, everyone with celiac disease is at risk of malnutrition.

How Common Is Celiac Disease?

You may think celiac disease is rare, but it's not! Worldwide, celiac disease is thought to occur in approximately 1 in 100 people. Studies have found it is most common in people of European descent, and apparently affects females about three times more often than males. There is some question about whether or not there is truly a higher prevalence in people of European descent, however. It could be that awareness is simply higher in that population, and they have, as a result, been more attentive to the diagnosis.

At one time it was thought that celiac disease was very rare in people of African and Asian descent, but recent studies indicate otherwise. It also occurs in other races, including North Africans, Arabs, and Slavic people. There are a variety of theories as to why celiac disease now seems more common in non-Europeans than previously. Perhaps at one time the incidence *was* lower due to a lack of gluten in the diet (i.e., wheat was not the most common grain in their diet), or perhaps cases were missed due to a lack of proper diagnosis. Then again, people in some countries may truly have a lower genetic susceptibility.

How Is Celiac Disease Diagnosed?

The procedures involved in diagnosing celiac disease are relatively straightforward and simple. Getting your doctor to perform those procedures and arrive at a diagnosis can be the tough part.

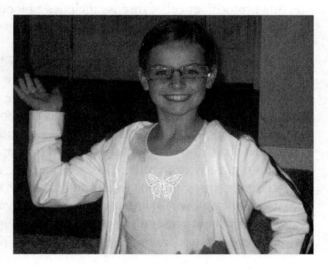

Most of us parents have consulted at *least* one pediatrician who brushed off our child's symptoms with a myriad of possible explanations: it's the antibiotics you're giving her for her ear infection; it's the flu; it's a reaction to something she ate. Whatever the excuse, the doctor hands you a sheet of paper with the B.R.A.T. diet and tells you to go home and wait it out. Diarrhea tends to be difficult to get rid of, they tell you. Some doctors even joke about how cute toddlers look with a big, round belly.

One problem is that many primary care pediatricians are not aware of celiac disease. Often they'll tell you that what you *perceive* to be problems—irritability, a distended belly, diarrhea—are "normal" for children. They may dismiss you with the patronizing advice that you should relax; nothing is wrong with your child. Even when asked directly about celiac disease, or told that celiac disease runs in the family, many pediatricians refuse to test for it. They may tell you that because your child is growing at a "normal" pace, is normal height and weight, she couldn't have celiac disease. This is *not* true!

If you reach an impasse with your pediatrician, you have four options:

1. Find a new doctor (we went through *four*, because our instincts told us that something was definitely wrong with our child, even though three doctors insisted that the symptoms should be ignored).
2. Educate your doctor (not all physicians are amenable to this, but if you have one who is, you're in good hands).
3. Ask to be referred to a specialist.

4. Trust that the doctor is right, and hope that your child is not being poisoned with every bite of cracker (and this is not truly an acceptable option).

If your child has symptoms, or even if there are no symptoms but celiac disease runs in your family, it is absolutely imperative that you insist on having your child tested. Change doctors if yours refuses, but don't stop until you succeed in finding someone who will test your child.

Testing Methods

Testing for celiac disease isn't an exact science—nor do "exact scientists" agree on protocol for some of the testing procedures available today. The most widely accepted testing protocol for celiac disease includes a blood test followed by an intestinal biopsy.

Blood Tests

Blood tests—also called *serological* tests—look for antibodies that the body produces when someone with a sensitivity or celiac disease eats gluten.

It's important to know that you have to be eating gluten for an extended length of time before having blood or biopsy testing done. If you don't eat gluten, or haven't eaten it for long enough, your body may not produce enough antibodies to show up on the blood tests, and the results will seem to show that you're "normal"—or "negative" for gluten sensitivity or celiac disease. The same goes for the biopsy (explained below). If you're not eating gluten, your small intestine will be healing or healed, and the biopsy will be negative for celiac disease even if you have it.

The most comprehensive panel of blood tests that you can get for gluten sensitivity and celiac disease includes five tests for antibodies:

◆ **tTG (anti-tissue transglutaminase)-IgA:** This test is very specific to celiac disease, meaning that if you have a positive tTG, it's very likely that you have celiac disease and not another condition.

◆ **EMA (anti-endomysial antibodies)-IgA:** This test is also specific to celiac disease. When it's positive, especially if tTG is positive too, it's extremely likely that you have celiac disease.

◆ **AGA (antigliadin antibodies)-IgA:** The antigliadin tests are less specific for celiac disease, and these antibodies sometimes show up in other diseases (including gluten sensitivity). AGA-IgA is useful when testing young symptomatic children, who don't always produce enough tTG or EMA for diagnostic purposes.
   ➤ AGA-IgA is also useful for monitoring compliance on the gluten-free diet (if it's still elevated after you've been gluten-free for several months, gluten may be sneaking into your diet). Some people feel that a positive AGA-IgA indicates gluten sensitivity.

◆ **AGA (antigliadin antibodies)-IgG:** This is another antigliadin test (like the preceding one) and is less specific to celiac disease, but it may be useful in detecting gluten sensitivity or leaky gut syndrome (see page 185). Also, if the IgG levels are highly positive and all the other tests are negative, that may signal that the patient is IgA-deficient (see the next point for more information on this), in which case the results of the other tests are erroneous.

◆ **Total serum IgA (total serum, immunoglobulin A):** A significant portion of the population is IgA-deficient, meaning their IgA production is always lower than normal. This is normal for them, and in most cases doesn't affect their health. Three of the four tests above are IgA-based (the only one that isn't IgA-based is antigliadin IgG), so in someone who's IgA-deficient, results of those three tests would be falsely low. By measuring total serum IgA, doctors can determine whether a patient is IgA-deficient and can compensate when reading the results of the three IgA-based tests. In other words, someone can be IgA deficient and have gluten sensitivity or celiac disease, but it complicates interpretation of tests.

Any lab can draw the blood, as long as you have an order from a doctor, registered nurse, chiropractor, or other health care practitioner allowed to order blood draws.

Follow-up antibody testing can be important in making sure you're not letting any gluten sneak into your diet. Most doctors recommend a follow-up blood test six months or a year after a diagnosis of celiac disease (and after presumably going on a strict gluten-free diet). If antibodies are still elevated at that time, you'll need to take a closer look at your diet and maybe see a dietitian who is knowledgeable about the GF diet to see what might be the culprit.

The "Gold Standard" for Diagnosing Celiac Disease: Endoscopy/Biopsy

Most physicians agree that the most accurate form of diagnosis is a series of intestinal endoscopies to biopsy the small intestine. Your child will be sedated, either with "conscious sedation" or, more likely, "unconscious sedation" (general anesthesia). While there are some risks inherent in anesthesia itself, general anesthesia is a safer way to perform an endoscopy because your child is completely relaxed.

The pediatric gastroenterologist usually does the actual procedure. An anesthesiologist is also present. A tube (endoscope) is inserted through the mouth, and threaded through the throat and stomach to the small intestine. The doctor is able to see what she's doing because there is a video camera on the endoscope. Once the endoscope reaches the small intestine, the doctor clips off several tissue samples, and sends them to a lab for a biopsy. The lab inspects the villi to see if they have flattened out (mucosal atrophy), or are blunted. The biopsy itself is not painful, because there are no pain-sensitive nerves inside the small intestine. Your child's throat may, however, be slightly sore afterwards.

Generally, the test is done first while your child is still very sick with symptoms. It is important that your child is still on a gluten-containing diet at the time of the endoscopy. The expectation at that time is to see blunted, atrophied villi.

If the villi are, in fact, damaged, then it is presumed that there is a strong possibility of celiac disease. Your child is put on a gluten-free diet for several (usually three to six) months. In some cases, a second biopsy is then performed (with the expectation that improvement in the villi will be seen).

Years ago, physicians generally recommended a third biopsy, for final confirmation. Today many doctors stop at the first or second biopsy and consider the diagnosis confirmed. However, your doctor may want to do a third biopsy, usually referred to as the "challenge." The challenge involves putting the child back on gluten for a period of time (generally a month or two), and doing a third biopsy (expecting to see damaged villi again). Challenges are not performed very often any more. If your doctor recommends one, be sure to ask him why. If he is questioning the diagnosis, ask him whether he reviewed the original biopsy. There is some evidence that challenges may actually be harmful to children.

While a biopsy *is* still considered the "gold standard" in diagnosing celiac disease, it does involve risks. There is a slight chance of internal injury, such as perforation of the bowel or excessive bleeding. Also, the sample of villi is small, and may not be representative of the entire small intestine. Furthermore, it can be difficult to obtain a good sample and some physicians may not be as skilled as others. Interpretation of the results can be subjective, as well. And finally, a "false negative" result can occur. In other words, a biopsy that comes back negative for celiac disease does not necessarily mean the patient doesn't have celiac disease. It's important to follow your instinct, and to press further with your doctor when you feel it is warranted. And be sure to request that the biopsy get sent to a pathologist experienced in diagnosing gastrointestinal disorders.

Stool Tests

At least one lab does home stool-testing for gluten sensitivity, microscopic colitis, genetic susceptibility, and several other gastrointestinal conditions. Like the blood test, the stool test looks for the immune system's reactions to gluten by detecting the presence of AGA and tTG antibodies.

The lab sends you a convenient container, and then you just do your business in it and send it back by overnight mail.

The most established lab doing this testing in the United States is EnteroLab, which claims the stool test is more sensitive than the blood test. In fact, a recent study showed that stool tests were actually more accurate in a positive diagnosis of celiac disease than blood tests.

EnteroLab asserts that because the immune response to food in gluten-sensitive individuals takes place in the intestine, antibodies are easily detectable in the stool, even before they're detectable in the blood. Therefore, people with slight sensitivities or people in the early phases of gluten sensitivity show an antibody response in stool testing, even if they don't show a response in blood tests.

This lab claims these advantages:

◆ The test is noninvasive.
◆ You don't need a doctor's involvement.
◆ The test is more sensitive than a blood test.
◆ You don't need to have eaten gluten recently for the test to be accurate.

Although stool testing certainly has some exciting and promising implications and offers some logistical advantages over the other testing methods, it is not yet considered a standard diagnostic tool for celiac disease.

Saliva Testing

There's a new saliva-based home-testing kit called MyCeliacID that does genetic testing for celiac disease. You order a kit online, and then just spit in the tube and send it back. Within a matter of days, you have your results. This is a highly specific test that looks for "risk stratification," meaning it can not only tell you if you do or don't have celiac disease, but how likely you are to get it. The table looks like this:

DQ Genotype	Increased Risk Over General Population	Relative Risk
DQ2 Homozygous	31x	Extremely High
DQ2 / other high risk gene	16x	Very High
DQ2 / DQ8	14x	Very High
DQ8 Homozygous	10x	High
DQ2 Heterozygous	10x	High
DQ8 Heterozygous	2x	Moderate
DQ2 / other low risk gene	<1x	Low
DQ2 negative / DQ8 negative	<0.1x	Extremely Low

The test is available at www.myceliacid.com.

Genetic Tests

Genetic tests can determine whether someone has the genes associated with celiac disease. Genetic testing can be done by blood or stool tests or a new saliva home test.

Genetic testing is valuable for ruling out celiac disease, because if your body doesn't produce either the protein HLA-DQ2 or HLA-DQ8, there's a 99 percent chance you don't have celiac disease. The test isn't valuable for predicting who will get celiac disease, though, because lots of people have these genes and never develop it.

It's important to note that for any type of genetic testing for celiac disease, you do not have to be on a gluten-containing diet for results to be accurate. You can be gluten-free—for any period of time—and the results will be the same.

Getting Siblings Tested

There is about a 30 percent chance that if one of your children has celiac disease, brothers and sisters will also have the condition, so it is especially important to have them tested. It doesn't matter how old the siblings are, as long as they're eating a gluten-containing diet.

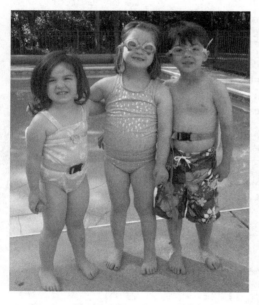

If you have a baby in addition to a child who has been diagnosed with celiac disease, it is a good idea to keep the baby gluten-free for the first year of her life. The question of whether or not nursing mothers can pass gluten through their breast milk has been debated for years. Recent studies seem to indicate that gluten is not, in fact, passed from a nursing mother to her baby. However, if there is reason to suspect that your baby might have celiac disease (because it runs in the family), it would be safest for the nursing mother to avoid gluten until the baby has been weaned. You should also know that many formulas are gluten-free, including the soy-based, lactose-free varieties (be sure to check with the manufacturer for sure).

Once your baby is a year old, slowly and selectively begin to add gluten to the diet, watching for any of the "classic" symptoms. (See the beginning of this chapter for a list of these symptoms.) Of course, if there are any indications of gastrointestinal distress or abnormalities, see your pediatrician and ask for a referral to a pediatric gastroenterologist. If, however, your child has been eased onto a completely "normal" (gluten-containing) diet with no symptoms whatsoever, you can assume that it is *likely* (but not for sure) that she does not have celiac disease. Even so, it is a good idea to have a serum antibody test done by age three or so, even if symptoms are not apparent.

Other People Who Should Be Tested

People with Conditions That Carry a Higher Risk of Celiac Disease

Even if they do not have any relatives diagnosed with celiac disease, people with the following conditions should be tested for celiac disease. This is true even if they exhibit none of the "classic" gastrointestinal symptoms.

- Type 1 diabetes mellitus
- Any other autoimmune disorder
- Down syndrome
- Cystic fibrosis
- Chronic active hepatitis
- Scleroderma
- Sjogren syndrome
- Raynaud syndrome
- Addison's disease
- Myasthenia gravis
- Rheumatoid arthritis
- Epilepsy or cerebral calcifications

People with the above conditions are more likely to have celiac disease than other people. These conditions do not necessarily *cause* celiac disease, but for some reason the conditions are associated with an increased risk of having celiac disease. For example, studies of people with Down syndrome have found incidences of celiac disease ranging between 5 and 16 percent.

I am 8 years old and I was diagnosed with celiac disease about 3 years ago. I think I had it longer because I always had problems with stomach aches, but no one ever knew it until my mom took me to a special doctor. I am glad that there are now more people discovering what celiac disease means/is. Now there are a lot of new great foods and now restaurants are taking care of it. Besides celiac disease I was just diagnosed with diabetes. It is hard living with both, but every day is what we choose to make of it, so let's handle a great life with celiac disease.

—Kathryn P., age 8

People with Conditions That Can Be Caused by Celiac Disease

People with the following conditions should also be tested for celiac disease. In these cases, celiac disease itself can be what causes the conditions:

- Selective IgA deficiency
- Unexplained anemia
- Deficiency in folic acid and other vitamins/minerals/nutrients
- Infertility
- Osteoporosis
- Growth retardation, short stature, failure to thrive
- Delayed puberty in children and adolescents

What Is Dermatitis Herpetiformis?

Dermatitis herpetiformis (DH) is a "sister" to celiac disease. Everyone with DH has celiac disease, but their primary symptoms—a very severe rash on their skin—are external. Internally, gluten usually wreaks the same havoc on the small intestine as it does in people with celiac disease. Seventy to eighty percent of people with DH have coexisting damage in the intestine.

DH is characterized by blistering, intensely itchy skin. Often it is initially misdiagnosed as eczema, but DH does not respond to eczema medications. The rash is found on the elbows, buttocks, knees, back, face, and/or scalp, and is usually symmetrical, meaning that it occurs in a mirror image from left to right.

DH is diagnosed by a small skin biopsy taken at the blister site. If IgA (immunoglobulin A) is present (see page 175), it confirms that there has been a reaction to the ingestion of gluten, and DH is the probable diagnosis. The treatment is a strict gluten-free diet.

People with Conditions That May Be Associated with Celiac Disease

It has been hypothesized that the disorders listed below *may* be associated with an increased incidence of celiac disease, but no direct links to celiac disease have been proven.

- ◆ Autism
- ◆ Attention deficit disorder (ADD)
- ◆ Multiple sclerosis (MS)
- ◆ Lactose intolerance
- ◆ Fibromyalgia
- ◆ ITP (Immune Thrombocytopenic Purpura)

Some people with these conditions may improve when put on a strict gluten-free diet, while others show no change. Because these underlying conditions are serious in nature, you should always advise your pediatrician of your intent to experiment with the GF diet. In addition to monitoring your child's health, your doctor may also provide valuable input that would help you measure the results of the diet more effectively.

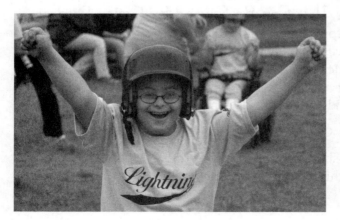

Remember that if you plan to test for the presence of anti-gluten antibodies, your child must be eating gluten. So, if you think you'll want the testing done and are interested in trying the diet, get the antibody test done *before* eliminating gluten from your child's diet.

The Consequences of Misdiagnosis or a Missed Diagnosis

If you don't get diagnosed—or get misdiagnosed—you're most likely going to continue to eat gluten. That's dangerous territory. There are many conditions that can develop if you or your child has celiac disease and continues to eat gluten. Some of these are due to the malnourishment that occurs with celiac disease; other conditions arise because they go hand-in-hand with celiac disease. Many of them are irreversible. You don't want to take a chance of developing these conditions just because there was a misdiagnosis—or a missed one.

How Is Celiac Disease Treated?

This is the beauty of celiac disease. After diagnosis, a strict gluten-free diet will be prescribed. Then you can expect your child to improve immediately! Depending upon the severity of the symptoms before diagnosis, you will see a child who is remarkably happier, more content and energetic, and has a better appetite. The bloated belly will slowly disappear, diarrhea should subside within a couple of weeks, and gas, cramping, and general discomfort will be a thing of the past. Growth, if previously affected, will increase quickly.

After a few weeks on the gluten-free diet, most people find that their energy levels increase and that they begin to "feel better" overall. Within a matter of months, you'll see dramatic improvement!

> *Even though I'm 17 and almost done with high school, I still remember when my mom, dad, and I realized that I had a gluten sensitivity. When I was taken off of gluten, my bloating, dark circles under my eyes, and winter earaches were all gone. I started to fill out and gain weight faster, and as a plus, some, if not all, of my ADD/ADHD symptoms diminished. Is my life over since I can't eat regular foods? No. It's just started. I can still eat out and go to parties, balls, and graduation parties with my friends and family—we just accommodate for me.*
>
> —Natalie J., age 17

23

Autism and the Gluten-Free/ Casein-Free Diet

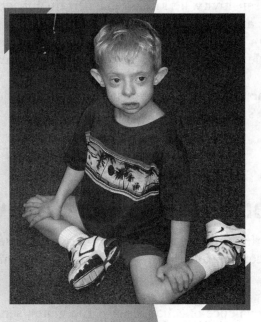

Autism is a developmental disorder that usually appears in the first few years of life. Kids on the autism spectrum engage in a variety of unusual behaviors, usually related to thought process, sensory stimulation, language, and social skills.

If you know or suspect that your child is on the autism spectrum, there are volumes of reputable reading materials available, and chances are you've already taken a deep dive into them. You're no doubt well aware that old-school thinking was that nothing much could be done for kids with autism. But today's prognosis is far more optimistic.

One of the most exciting areas of discussion centers around the gluten-free/casein-free (GFCF) diet. Most of what I discuss in this chapter has yet to be proven or disproven, because there just hasn't been a lot of research in this area. It's understandable that there aren't better studies yet; it's nearly impossible to set a double-blind, placebo-controlled study involving diet unless the kids being studied are in an inpatient setting (which would influence behavior and skew results). So for now, we have hypotheses and anecdotal evidence. However, I personally have heard thousands of stories of kids with autism improving (sometimes dramatically) on a GFCF diet, and I'll tell you, they're nothing short of miraculous.

We Do Know That Gluten Affects Behavior

It's widely accepted that gluten has an effect on behavior for kids with gluten sensitivities. Behavioral manifestations of celiac disease or gluten sensitivity include:
- Inability to concentrate or focus
- Attention deficit disorder (ADD) and attention-deficit/hyperactivity disorder (ADHD) type behaviors
- Depression, bipolar disorder, schizophrenia, and mood disorders
- Irritability and anxiety
- Lack of motivation

The nutrition chapter talks about nutritional deficiencies that can arise when someone has celiac disease or gluten sensitivity. It's known that certain nutrients—including folate (folic acid), vitamin D, and essential fatty acids—are linked to moods, sex drive, sleeping patterns, and your appetite. It's no wonder, then, that the nutritional deficiencies that arise in people with celiac disease and gluten sensitivity can affect behavior.

But that's jumping back to celiac disease and gluten sensitivity. What does this have to do with autism? Ah, now that's a tangled web.

The Relationship among Autism, Celiac Disease, and Gluten Sensitivity

There have been many studies that indicate relationships between these conditions—but again, nothing that has been clearly proven—or disproven. Here are some important points to consider:

- Autism carries with it a higher prevalence of celiac disease and gluten sensitivity. In fact, some studies show that kids with autism have a three-times higher rate of celiac disease than kids in the general population. But is that because people with autism are more likely to have celiac disease? Or because people with celiac disease are more likely to have autism?

◆ Because some of the symptoms of celiac disease and gluten sensitivity can mimic some of those of autism, how do we know for sure whether a child's autistic symptoms are actually caused by autism? What if, at least in some cases, the child actually has celiac disease? If so, it's no wonder that a gluten-free diet would improve behaviors.

◆ If research some day shows that autism is separate from celiac disease, it is still similar in the fact that it responds well (sometimes in the case of autism) to a gluten-free diet.

◆ Could the malabsorption of nutrients that is characteristic of celiac disease actually result in a deficiency of important neurotransmitters in the brain, and therefore create autistic behaviors?

◆ What about the other way around? Could it be that in at least some cases when children are diagnosed with celiac disease at a very early age the gluten-free diet prevents autistic behaviors from emerging?

◆ Autism is known to be related to autoimmune diseases (celiac disease is an autoimmune disease). A recent study done in Denmark showed that children whose mothers have autoimmune diseases are up to three times more likely to have autism. The study looked at kids whose moms had type-1 diabetes, rheumatoid arthritis, and celiac disease. The risk of having kids with autism was 2 times higher for those with diabetes; 1.5 times higher for those with rheumatoid arthritis, and more than 3 times higher for those with celiac disease.

Anecdotal evidence shows us that when some people with autism go gluten-free (and casein-free) their autistic behaviors diminish or disappear completely. Could it be that they were never autistic? That their celiac symptoms simply made them appear to be autistic, so once they eliminated gluten from their diets, they returned to a "normal" state? Or is it more likely that the gluten-free diet sometimes really does help improve the behaviors of autism?

Leaky Gut Syndrome

One of the more common associations between celiac disease and autism has been well documented: leaky gut syndrome. Leaky gut is a condition in which things such as toxins that shouldn't be able to make their way out of the intestinal walls and into the bloodstream are able to do so. People with celiac disease and gluten sensitivity have leaky gut syndrome—that's why gluten, a large molecule that shouldn't be able to get through the intestinal walls and into the bloodstream, is able to do so.

Kids with autism have a high incidence of leaky gut syndrome. But which comes first? Does the leaky gut (maybe a result of gluten sensitivity or celiac disease?) allow gluten and other toxins to get into the bloodstream and then cause autistic behaviors?

Or do people with autism develop celiac disease more often because they have leaky gut? Or is there absolutely no connection whatsoever?

No one knows yet. But we do know that lots of parents are claiming success with the gluten-free/casein-free dietary intervention protocol for treating autism.

The Hypothesis Behind Why the Diet Works

The theory is that some people with autism may metabolize gluten and casein (casein is the protein found in milk) into the form of an opiate—similar to the type of opiate that's found in heroin. Basically, the idea is that when they eat these proteins, they're getting a high from them and, at the same time, they're becoming addicted.

The specific theory is called the Opioid Excess Theory of Autism, first presented by Kalle Reichelt in 1991. In all people, gluten and casein are broken down to peptides called gliadinomorphin and casomorphine, respectively. In nonautistic people, these peptides are broken down further into constituent amino acids—but in autistic people (the theory goes), they're not.

In people with autism, the theory contends, these peptides cross through the intestine, into the bloodstream, and ultimately into the brain. The question is, how do such large molecules get into the bloodstream? Through the leaky gut—and therein lies one of the connections with celiac disease and gluten sensitivity.

Because their chemical structures are similar to that of morphine, a powerful opiate, gliadinomorphin and casomorphine are suspected of causing an opiate effect. This "high" may account for traits common in children with autism, such as repetitive body movements (for instance, finger-flicking in front of their eyes, spinning, and head-banging), as well as being withdrawn and having a fascination with parts of objects (like fixating on one part of a toy rather than the toy itself). Also typical of opiate users is the distress people with autism often feel when there are small changes in their environment or routine.

According to the Opioid Excess theory, the addiction that kids with autism experience is similar to that of a drug addict, but what they are physiologically addicted to is gluten and casein. Many of these children already have limited diets, and often those diets are limited to breads and milk products—gluten and casein. It's a combination of this possible addiction and the child's resistance to trying new foods that can make it tough to eliminate these foods from the diet.

It may not be hard-core evidence, but the proof is in the pee. Sure enough, many people with autism (who are not on GFCF diets) have elevated levels of these gluten- and casein-related peptides in their urine, whereas most nonautistic people do not.

See Ya, Soy?

Some people believe that you should eliminate soy as well as gluten and casein to see the most improvement in kids with autism. Sometimes the soy elimination is incorporated into the dietary protocol as a two- to three-week no-soy trial, and parents keep a daily food journal that documents their child's behavioral changes during the trial period. Then soy is rotated back into the diet for every meal and snack for one day—and then four days of no soy again.

During the trial period, notation should be made of changes in activity level, discomfort, sleep abnormalities, and skin or bowel problems. If the child has a strong intolerance, it will show up quickly. If there aren't any reactions during the trial, it's probably okay to reintroduce soy on a regular basis.

What You Should Expect

Because results are so variable, you should take a wait-and-see approach. Those who do see improvement on the GFCF diet sometimes see improvement as fast as within a week. Others see improvements within a year, and still others, of course, see no improvement whatsoever.

The changes that parents note are variable, too. Some kids start sleeping through the night when they couldn't before. Others become more verbal and interactive. And still others become completely "normalized" on the diet.

Remember, though, that the connection between these improvements and the GFCF diet are anecdotal. Also bear in mind that—assuming the child is receiving other treatments for autism such as educational interventions, speech therapy, or medications—it can be next to impossible to determine which improvements are due to which treatment.

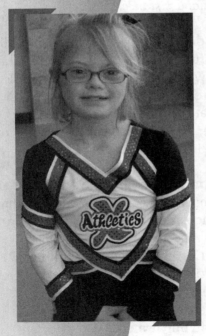

24 Your Legal Rights and Benefits

Throughout this book, I have emphasized that celiac disease, gluten sensitivity, and related conditions are something that you and your child can not only learn to live with, but also to thrive with. I have focused on ways to make your child's experiences as much like any other child's as possible, and certainly have not suggested that these conditions, in and of themselves, are disabling in any way.

Still, there are a few instances when it *may* benefit your child to know about some of the federal laws and regulations relating to children with disabilities or serious health concerns. This is especially the case if your child happens to have a bona fide disability (such as Down syndrome, epilepsy, or attention-deficit hyperactivity disorder) in addition to celiac disease. Please note that these guidelines as far as dietary restrictions are concerned are clearly delineated for celiac disease, but they are not so clear for gluten sensitivity. We will, for that reason, refer to celiac disease in this chapter; other conditions will need to be addressed on a personal, case-by-case basis.

At School

If your child with celiac disease attends public school, there are two federal laws that may be relevant:

1. Section 504 of the Rehabilitation Act of 1973, which applies to most students with a diagnosis of celiac disease, and
2. The Individuals with Disabilities Education Act (IDEA), which applies only to students who have a disability that has an "educational impact" on their ability to learn (e.g., students with celiac disease who also have a disability such as Down syndrome, autism, epilepsy, or ADHD).

Section 504 of the Rehabilitation Act of 1973 *

Section 504 of the Rehabilitation Act of 1973 states:
"No otherwise qualified individual with handicaps in the United States…shall solely by reason of her or his handicap, be excluded from the participation in, be denied the benefits of, or be subjected to discrimination under any program or activity receiving federal financial assistance…."

In other words, the law prohibits discrimination on the basis of disability in any program or activity receiving federal funds. Since public schools all receive federal funding, the law ensures that students with disabilities receive equal access to a public education. Private schools and childcare centers that receive any public funding must also comply with this law and its regulations.

For your child with celiac disease, the main protection this law offers is to prohibit discrimination when she is eating in a public school cafeteria.

Section 504 defines a person with a disability as any person who:
◆ has a physical or mental impairment that substantially limits one or more major life activities such as caring for oneself, performing manual tasks, walking, seeing, hearing, speaking, breathing, learning, **eating,** sleeping, concentrating, thinking, and working (the list is not exhaustive and many activities or functions not listed can still be considered major life activities);
◆ has a record of such an impairment; or
◆ is regarded as having such an impairment.

---

* The following information has been adapted from "Students with Food Allergies: What Do the Laws Say?" published by the Food Allergy Network, Fairfax, VA.

Related Aids and Services

Under Section 504, a school district must consider the individual needs of a child with disabilities and provide special education and related aids and services to enable that child to attend school and benefit from the program. These requirements may include the following:

- ◆ health services, including the administration of medication;
- ◆ related and supplementary aids and services for students with disabilities in order to enable them to benefit from regular or special education—for example, readers for blind students or menu information or ingredient substitution for students with food allergies.

Free and Appropriate Public Education

Section 504 requires federally funded public elementary and secondary education programs to provide a "free and appropriate public education" to students, regardless of the severity of the student's disability.

"Free education" means the parents will incur no costs. A school cannot charge parents, for example, for the cost of food or ingredient substitutions, or other services in the cafeteria to a student with dietary restrictions.

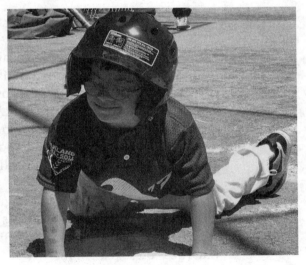

"Appropriate education" means:

- ◆ A student with a disability must be educated with nondisabled students to the extent that it is appropriate for that student.
- ◆ A student with a disability must receive access to educational opportunities or extracurricular activities equal to that provided to students without disabilities. For example, students cannot be excluded from field trips, eating in the cafeteria, or class projects because of a food allergy or celiac disease.

How Do Celiac Kids Fit into Section 504?

Section 504 requires meals to be modified for children who have a "handicapping condition" that restricts their diet, yet Section 504 does not outline how this is to be done. However, it mandates that the United States Department of Agriculture (USDA) issue instructions for State Departments of Education.

The USDA responded to this mandate by including this information in the National School Lunch Act (NSLA). Under the NSLA, public schools must provide special diets for:

◆ Students on an "Individualized Education Program" (IEP) who have a physician's statement of need. (Children who have Down syndrome, autism, epilepsy, or another developmental disability in addition to celiac disease would qualify under this criterion. See the next section.)

◆ Students with a food allergy or medical condition requiring a special diet who are not on an IEP (e.g., celiac disease, PKU, diabetes,) with a physician's statement of need.

A physician's statement of need is required to obtain a special diet at school, and must be in the student's file. (Without a doctor's note, the school can deny your request, since not all food allergies are life-threatening.) The physician's statement must include:

◆ the student's disability (celiac disease),
◆ the major life activity affected by the disability, and
◆ the foods to be omitted or substituted.

It's a good idea to take the following steps if you want your child to use the school's food service:

1. Obtain a statement of need that says: "(Child's name) is to be provided with a gluten-free diet per dietitian's guidelines secondary to celiac disease. Gluten will cause malabsorption and malnutrition, which will interfere with school participation." This should be written on the physician's stationery or a prescription pad, and signed by the physician.
2. Obtain a list of safe and unsafe foods from a reliable source.
3. Ask the food service staff who will review the menu to be certain it is gluten-free.
4. Ask if a registered dietitian will sign off on these menu modifications.
5. Provide a copy of the physician's statement and list of safe/unsafe foods for your child's file, the office staff, the classroom teacher(s), and the food service staff.
6. Also present this file to the school principal, and provide a copy to the school district office.

You should be aware that if the school district does not provide lunches to *any* children (there is no school lunch program in place), which may be the case in small, rural towns, the school cannot be required to provide a gluten-free diet to your child. Also remember that, in practice, it is often simpler to provide a homemade gluten-free lunch for your child to take to school.

The Individuals with Disabilities Education Act (IDEA)

The Individuals with Disabilities Education Act (IDEA) is a federal law that guarantees a free and appropriate education to all children who have disabilities that have an educational impact on their ability to learn at school. Specifically, it applies to children who have been diagnosed with:

- ◆ an intellectual disability (mental retardation)
- ◆ hearing impairments (including deafness)
- ◆ speech or language impairments
- ◆ visual impairments (including blindness)
- ◆ serious emotional disturbance
- ◆ orthopedic impairments
- ◆ autism
- ◆ tramatic brain injury
- ◆ other health impairments (including epilepsy, diabetes, and attention deficit disorders)
- ◆ specific learning disabilities
- ◆ developmental delay (an optional category used in some states for children aged 3–9 who have not yet received a formal disability diagnosis but have significant delays in physical, cognitive, communication, or social/emotional skills).

As mentioned above, the law does *not* apply to children who only have celiac disease, but does apply to children who have celiac disease in addition to one of the qualifying disabilities above.

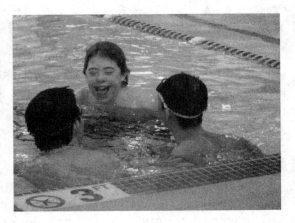

Children who qualify under IDEA receive an Individualized Education Program (IEP). For children three and older, the IEP is a written plan that describes long-term goals for, as well as the services that will be provided, to help the child reach those goals, and the setting where the services will be provided. An IEP is developed by a team consisting of school personnel, parents, and the child herself, if she chooses to participate.

It is beyond the scope of this book to explain the basics of qualifying for services under IDEA, or to go into detail about writing good IEPs. You should know, however, that if your child has an IEP because she has Down syndrome, autism, or another disability, the IEP can include goals and services related to helping her learn to manage her celiac disease.

Remember, your child's IEP will be *individualized* to her needs and abilities, so it is impossible to list goals that would be appropriate for all children who have celiac disease in addition to another disability. Here are a few examples, though, that might be appropriate for some children:

◆ If the class as a whole has a unit on nutrition, a goal for your child might be to understand how gluten fits into the food pyramid, and what gluten-free substitutions can be made for foods listed on the pyramid.

◆ If your child is receiving speech therapy as a related service, a goal might be for her to learn to request gluten-free items in the cafeteria, either verbally or by using some kind of alternative and augmentative system (pictures of "safe" foods on a key ring, voice output computer, etc.).

◆ For an older child who is learning functional skills, goals could be related to learning to read and to use a list of "safe" foods and ingredients when shopping or preparing foods.

◆ A child who continually tries to eat her classmates' (gluten-containing) food in the cafeteria or during school parties could have a plan for positive behavioral support in this area written into her IEP.

It is important to note that any student covered by IDEA is also covered by Section 504. She would therefore be able to obtain the same modifications to the school lunch program described above, as long as she had a doctor's prescription stating that need.

The Americans with Disabilities Act

The Americans with Disabilities Act (ADA) takes up where Section 504 of the Rehabilitation Act leaves off. Whereas Section 504 only prohibits discrimination against people with disabilities by agencies receiving federal funding, the ADA extends protections into many more areas of public life.

The ADA is divided into five titles or sections. For people with celiac disease, the sections with the most relevance are Title 1 (Employment) and Title III (Public Accommodations).

Title I: Employment. This section prohibits employers from discriminating against qualified individuals with disabilities during the application or hiring process, or when determining salary, benefits, or other aspects of employment. It prohibits employers from asking whether an applicant has a disability and refusing to hire someone solely because she has a disability, or because she is perceived as having a disability. If an employee tells her employer about her disability, however, then the employer must provide "reasonable accommodations" (modifications to the job) to help the employee succeed—provided the accommodation does not impose an "undue hardship" on the employer.

Title III: Public Accommodations. A public accommodation is a business, program, or agency that provides services or goods to the public. The ADA lists twelve categories of public accommodations, including: places of lodging (inns, hotels, motels); establishments serving food or drink; places of exhibition or entertainment (movie theaters, stadiums, concert halls); sales or retail establishments (stores of all kinds, shopping centers); places of public display or collection (museums, libraries); schools serving students of all ages; places of exercise or recreation (gyms, health spas, bowling alleys); places that provide testing services. *(Facilities run by religious entities and private clubs are excepted.)*

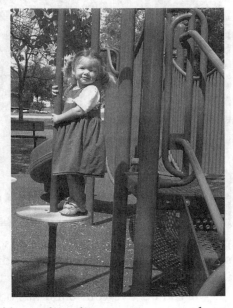

Under ADA, individuals with disabilities are entitled to "full and equal enjoyment of the goods, services, facilities, privileges, advantages, or accommodations" of any place of public accommodation.

For your child, this section of the ADA means that she should not be denied the opportunity to go anywhere or do anything because of her celiac disease. For example, a childcare center may be required to change its policy regarding sharing foods, or a summer camp may need to make gluten-free menu items available as a way of accommodating your child's special diet. Likewise, it is against the law for a restaurant to refuse to serve people who require special diets due to a disability.

Who Is Covered by the ADA?

The ADA defines "disability" very broadly. Under this law, an individual is protected from discrimination if:

◆ She is perceived as having a disability. For instance, you and your child may not consider celiac disease the least bit disabling, but if an employer or other individual discriminates against your child because *he* thinks celiac disease is a disability, your child would be covered by the law.

◆ She is related to, or associated with, someone who has a disability. For example, it would be against the law for an employer to refuse to hire or promote you solely because he thinks you are the parent of a child with a disability, and that your childcare duties might be too time consuming.

◆ She actually has a disability that substantially limits a major life activity—to include, but not limited to caring for herself, performing manual tasks, walking, seeing, hearing, speaking, breathing, learning, working, thinking, concentrating, and interacting with other people.

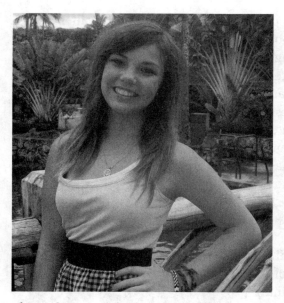

In reality, most families of children with celiac disease will likely never need to use the ADA to obtain the accommodations their child needs. Most restaurants are more than happy to serve people who need gluten-free meals. (Note that they are not required under the ADA to list GF options on their menu, but if asked to modify an existing menu choice to make it gluten free, they would be expected to comply under ADA.) The vast majority of daycare centers, schools, and recreation departments will willingly work with you to handle your child's special dietary needs, and few employers would even dream of discriminating against an employee because she has celiac disease. However, on the off chance that you encounter someone who does perceive celiac disease as a disability worthy of discrimination, it is good to know that the ADA protects your child.

If you believe your child has been discriminated against under Titles II or III of the ADA, you can contact The U.S. Department of Justice, Civil Rights Division, Coordination and Review Section (800-514-0301; 800-514-0383 TTY). You may also bring a lawsuit against any business or program that you feel has discriminated against you or your child under ADA.

Income Tax Deductions

Considering what it can cost to keep your child on a gluten-free diet, it would be nice if you could write some of the extra cost off, wouldn't it? In fact, the Internal Revenue Service does allow income tax deductions for people with dietary restrictions. There are four areas that qualify.

1. The law says that the *additional* expense of special dietary products may be deducted. For instance, if a "regular" loaf of bread costs $2.50 and a gluten-free loaf of bread costs $4.50, the $2.00 difference may be deducted. Special gluten-free mixes, pastas, and any other items also qualify.
2. The full cost of special items needed for a gluten-free diet may be deducted. The cost of xanthan gum (methyl cellulose), for instance, may be deducted, because it is used in gluten-free home-baked items, but is completely different from anything used in an ordinary recipe.
3. If you make a special trip to a specialty store to purchase gluten-free foods, the actual cost of your transportation to and from the store is

deductible. If you are using your vehicle for the trip, you will need to check with the IRS for current mileage deduction amounts.

4. The full cost of postage or other delivery expenses on gluten-free purchases made by mail order are deductible.

The total amount of your deduction for gluten-free foods should be added to your other medical expenses that are reported on line 1 of Schedule A on form 1040 (for taxpayers who itemize deductions). Your expenses must exceed a certain percentage of your adjusted gross income for any of the amount to be deductible. Please check with the IRS to ensure that these tax laws are up to date.

If you are audited, you will need a letter from your doctor stating that your child has celiac disease and must adhere to a gluten-free diet for life. You will also need substantiation in the form of receipts, cash register tapes, or canceled checks for your gluten-free purchases, and a schedule showing how you computed your deductions for the gluten-free foods.

A Final Word from Danna

Whether you've already decided to put your child on a gluten-free diet or are still in the considering-all-your-options stage, I commend you for having an open mind and a commitment to your child's improved health.

If your child has been diagnosed with celiac disease, gluten sensitivity, autism, or any other condition that may benefit from being gluten-free—or even if he hasn't and you're doing this for other reasons—the gluten-free diet will be a great thing for your child.

The beauty of these conditions is that a natural, healthy diet will improve, if not fully restore, health. We're talking about conditions where no medications or surgical procedures are required to ensure a lifetime of happiness and good health! Keeping your child on a strict gluten-free diet is all it takes. Okay, the diet isn't always a piece of gluten-free cake, but the outcome can be remarkable—besides, understanding how to implement the diet is what this book is for. Remember, *deal with it—don't dwell on it!*

Best wishes for your child's optimum health and well-being.

Remember: ***Gluten-free's the way to be!***

Danna

Appendix

Safe and Forbidden Ingredients and Additives

This list is reprinted courtesy of Scott Adams (www.celiac.com)

SAFE LIST

Acacia Gum
Acesulfame K
Acesulfame Potassium
Acetanisole
Acetophenone
Acorn Quercus
Adipic Acid
Adzuki Bean
Agar
Agave
Albumen
Alcohol (Spirits—Specific Types)
Alfalfa
Algae
Algin
Alginate
Alginic Acid
Alkalized Cocoa
Allicin
Almond Nut
Alpha-amylase
Alpha-lactalbumin
Aluminum
Amaranth
Ambergris
Ammonium Hydroxide
Ammonium Phosphate
Ammonium Sulphate
Amylopectin
Amylose
Annatto
Annatto Color

Apple Cider Vinegar
Arabic Gum
Arrowroot
Artichokes
Artificial Butter Flavor
Artificial Flavoring
Ascorbic Acid
Aspartame (can cause IBS symptoms)
Aspartic Acid
Aspic
Astragalus Gummifer
Autolyzed Yeast Extract
Avena Sativia (Oats[3])
Avena Sativia Extract (from Oats[3])
Avidin
Azodicarbonamide
Baking Soda
Balsamic Vinegar
Beeswax
Beans
Bean, Adzuki
Bean, Hyacinth
Bean, Lentil
Bean, Mung
Bean Romano (Chickpea)
Bean Tepary
Benzoic acid
Besan (Chickpea)
Beta Glucan (from Oats[3])
Betaine
Beta Carotene
BHA
BHT
Bicarbonate of Soda

Biotin
Blue Cheese
Brown Sugar
Buckwheat
Butter (check additives)
Butyl Compounds
Butylated Hydroxyanisole
Calcium Acetate
Calcium Carbonate
Calcium Caseinate
Calcium Chloride
Calcium Disodium
Calcium Hydroxide
Calcium Lactate
Calcium Pantothenate
Calcium Phosphate
Calcium Propionate
Calcium Silicate
Calcium Sorbate
Calcium Stearate
Calcium Stearoyl Lactylate
Calcium Sulfate
Calrose
Camphor
Cane Sugar
Cane Vinegar
Canola (Rapeseed)
Canola Oil (Rapeseed Oil)
Caprylic Acid
Carageenan Chondrus Crispus
Carbonated Water
Carboxymethyl Cellulose
Carmine
Carnauba Wax
Carob Bean
Carob Bean Gum
Carob Flour
Carrageenan
Casein
Cassava Manihot Esculenta
Castor Oil
Catalase
Cellulose[1]

Cellulose Ether
Cellulose Gum
Cetyl Alcohol
Cetyl Stearyl Alcohol
Champagne Vinegar
Channa (Chickpea)
Chana Flour (Chickpea Flour)
Cheeses—(most, but check ingredients)
Chestnuts
Chickpea
Chlorella
Chocolate Liquor
Choline Chloride
Chromium Citrate
Chymosin
Citric Acid
Citrus Red No. 2
Cochineal
Cocoa
Cocoa Butter
Coconut
Coconut Vinegar
Collagen
Colloidal Silicon Dioxide
Confectioner's Glaze
Copernicia Cerifera
Copper Sulphate
Corn
Corn Flour
Corn Gluten
Corn Masa Flour
Corn Meal
Corn Starch
Corn Sugar
Corn Sugar Vinegar
Corn Syrup
Corn Syrup Solids
Corn Swetener
Corn Vinegar
Corn Zein
Cortisone
Cotton Seed
Cotton Seed Oil

Cowitch
Cowpea
Cream of Tartar
Crospovidone
Curds
Cyanocobalamin
Cysteine, L
Dal (Lentils)
D-Alpha-tocopherol
Dasheen Flour (Taro)
Dates
D-Calcium Pantothenate
Delactosed Whey
Demineralized Whey
Desamidocollagen
Dextran
Dextrose
Diglycerides
Dioctyl Sodium
Dioctyl Sodium Solfosuccinate
Dipotassium Phosphate
Disodium Guanylate
Disodium Inosinate
Disodium Phosphate
Distilled Alcohols
Distilled Vinegar
Distilled White Vinegar
Dutch Processed Cocoa
EDTA (Ethylenediaminetetraacetic Acid)
Eggs
Egg Yolks
Elastin
Ester Gum
Ethyl Alcohol
Ethylenediaminetetraacetic Acid
Ethyl Maltol
Ethyl Vanillin
Expeller Pressed Canola Oil
FD&C Blue No. 1 Dye
FD&C Blue No. 1 Lake
FD&C Blue No. 2 Dye
FD&C Blue No. 2 Lake
FD&C Green No. 3 Dye

FD&C Green No. 3 Lake
FD&C Red No. 3 Dye
FD&C Red No. 40 Dye
FD&C Red No. 40 Lake
FD&C Yellow No. 5 Dye
FD&C Yellow No. 6 Dye
FD&C Yellow No. 6 Lake
Ferric Orthophosphate
Ferrous Fumerate
Ferrous Gluconate
Ferrous Lactate
Ferrous Sulfate
Fish (fresh)
Flaked Rice
Flax
Folacin
Folate
Folic Acid-Folacin
Formaldehyde
Fructose
Fruit (including dried)
Fruit Vinegar
Fumaric Acid
Galactose
Garbanzo Beans
Gelatin
Glucoamylase
Gluconolactone
Glucose
Glucose Syrup
Glutamate (free)
Glutamic Acid
Glutamine (amino acid)
Glutinous Rice
Glutinous Rice Flour
Glycerides
Glycerin
Glycerol Monooleate
Glycol
Glycol Monosterate
Glycolic acid
Gram flour (chick peas)
Grape Skin Extract

Grits, Corn
Guar Gum
Gum Acacia
Gum Arabic
Gum Base
Gum Tragacanth
Hemp
Hemp Seeds
Herbs
Herb Vinegar
Hexanedioic Acid
High Fructose Corn Syrup
Hominy
Honey
Hops
Horseradish (Pure)
Hyacinth Bean
Hydrogen Peroxide
Hydrolyzed Caseinate
Hydrolyzed Meat Protein
Hydrolyzed Soy Protein
Hydroxypropyl Cellulose
Hydroxypropyl Methylcellulose
Hypromellose
Illepe
Inulin
Invert Sugar
Iodine
Iron Ammonium Citrate
Isinglass
Isolated Soy Protein
Isomalt
Job's Tears
Jowar (Sorghum)
Karaya Gum
Kasha (roasted buckwheat)
Keratin
K-Carmine Color
K-Gelatin
Koshihikari (rice)
Kudzu
Kudzu Root Starch
Lactalbumin Phosphate

Lactase
Lactic Acid
Lactitol
Lactose
Lactulose
Lanolin
Lard
L-cysteine
Lecithin
Lemon Grass
Lentils
Licorice
Licorice Extract
Lipase
L-leucine
L-lysine
L-methionine
Locust Bean Gum
L-tryptophan
Magnesium Carbonate
Magnesium Hydroxide
Magnesium Oxide
Maize
Maize Waxy
Malic Acid
Maltitol
Maltodextrin
Maltol
Manganese Sulfate
Manioc
Masa
Masa Flour
Masa Harina
Meat (fresh)
Medium Chain Triglycerides
Menhaden Oil
Methyl Cellulose[2]
Microcrystalline Cellulose
Micro-particulated Egg White Protein
Milk
Milk Protein Isolate
Millet
Milo (Sorghum)

Mineral Oil
Mineral Salts
Molybdenum Amino Acid Chelate
Mono and Diglycerides
Monocalcium Phosphate
Monoglycerides
Monopotassium Phosphate
Monosaccharides
Monosodium Glutamate (MSG)
Monostearates
MSG
Mung Bean
Musk
Mustard Flour
Myristic Acid
Natural Smoke Flavor
Niacin-Niacinamide
Neotame
Niacin
Niacinamide
Nitrates
Nitrous Oxide
Nonfat Milk
Nuts (except wheat, rye, & barley)
Nut, Acorn
Nut, Almond
Oats[3]
Oils and Fats
Oleic Acid
Oleoresin
Olestra
Oleyl Alcohol/Oil
Orange B
Oryzanol
Palmitic Acid
Pantothenic Acid
Papain
Paprika
Paraffin
Patially Hydrogenated Cottonseed Oil
Patially Hydrogenated Soybean Oil
Pea—Chick
Pea—Cow

Pea Flour
Pea Starch
Peanut Flour
Peanuts
Peas
Pectin
Pectinase
Peppermint Oil
Peppers
Pepsin
Peru Balsam
Petrolatum
PGPR (Polyglycerol Polyricinoleate)
Phenylalanine
Phosphoric Acid
Phosphoric Glycol
Pigeon Peas
Polenta
Polydextrose
Polyethylene Glycol
Polyglycerol
Polyglycerol Polyricinoleate (PGPR)
Polysorbates
Polysorbate 60
Polysorbate 80
Potassium Benzoate
Potassium Caseinate
Potassium Citrate
Potassium Iodide
Potassium Lactate
Potassium Matabisulphite
Potassium Sorbate
Potatoes
Potato Flour
Potato Starch
Povidone
Prinus
Pristane
Propolis
Propylene Glycol
Propylene Glycol Monosterate
Propyl Gallate
Protease

Psyllium
Pyridoxine Hydrochloride
Quinoa
Ragi
Raisin Vinegar
Rape
Recaldent
Reduced Iron
Rennet
Rennet Casein
Resinous Glaze
Reticulin
Riboflavin
Rice
Rice (Enriched)
Rice Flour
Rice Starch
Rice Syrup
Rice Vinegar
Ricinoleic Acid
Romano Bean (chickpea)
Rosematta
Rosin
Royal Jelly
Saccharin
Saffron
Sago
Sago Flour
Sago Palm
Sago Starch
Saifun (bean threads)
Salt
Seaweed
Seed—Sesame
Seed—Sunflower
Seeds (except wheat, rye, & barley)
Shea
Sherry Vinegar
Silicon Dioxide
Soba (be sure it's 100% buckwheat)
Sodium Acetate
Sodium Acid Pyrophosphate
Sodium Alginate

Sodium Ascorbate
Sodium Benzoate
Sodium Caseinate
Sodium Citrate
Sodium Erythrobate
Sodium Hexametaphosphate
Sodium Lactate
Sodium Lauryl Sulfate
Sodium Metabisulphite
Sodium Nitrate
Sodium Phosphate
Sodium Polyphosphate
Sodium Silaco Aluminate
Sodium Stannate
Sodium Stearoyl Lactylate
Sodium Sulphite
Sodium Tripolyphosphate
Sorbic Acid
Sorbitan Monostearate
Sorbitol-Mannitol
   (can cause IBS symptoms)
Sorghum
Sorghum Flour
Soy
Soybean
Soy Lecithin
Soy Protein
Soy Protein Isolate
Spices (pure)
Spirit Vinegar
Spirits (Specific Types)
Stearamide
Stearamine
Stearates
Stearic Acid
Stearyl Lactate
Stevia
Succotash (corn and beans)
Sucralose
Sucrose
Sulfites
Sulfosuccinate
Sulfur Dioxide

Sunflower Seed
Sweet Chestnut Flour
Tagatose
Tallow
Tapioca
Tapioca Flour
Tapioca Starch
Tara Gum
Taro
Tarro
Tarrow Root
Tartaric Acid
Tartrazine
TBHQ is Tetra or Tributylhydroquinone
Tea
Tea-Tree Oil
Teff
Teff Flour
Tepary Bean
Textured Vegetable Protein
Thiamin Hydrochloride
Thiamine Hydrochloride
Thiamine Mononitrate
Titanium Dioxide
Tofu (Soy Curd)
Tolu Balsam
Torula Yeast
Tragacanth
Tragacanth Gum
Triacetin
Tricalcium Phosphate
Trypsin
Turmeric (Kurkuma)
TVP

Tyrosine
Urad/Urid Beans
Urad/Urid Dal (peas) Vegetables
Urad/Urid flour
Urd
Vanilla Extract
Vanilla Flavoring
Vanillin
Vinegar (All except Malt)
Vinegars (Specific Types)
Vitamin A (retinol)
Vitamin A Palmitate
Vitamin B1
Vitamin B2
Vitamin B6
Vitamin B12
Vitamin D
Vitamin E Acetate
Waxy Maize
Whey
Whey Protein Concentrate
Whey Protein Isolate
White Vinegar
Wild Rice
Wines
Wine Vinegars (& Balsamic)
Xanthan Gum
Xylitol
Yam Flour
Yeast
Yogurt (plain, unflavored)
Zinc Oxide
Zinc Sulfate

1. Cellulose is a carbohydrate polymer of D-glucose. It is the structural material of plants, such as wood in trees. It contains no gluten protein.
2. Methyl cellulose is a chemically modified form of cellulose that makes a good substitute for gluten in rice-based breads, etc.
3. Recent research indicates that oats may be safe for people on gluten-free diets, although many people may also have an additional, unrelated intolerance to them. Cross contamination with wheat is also a factor that you need to consider before choosing to include oats in your diet.

FORBIDDEN LIST

Abyssinian Hard (Wheat triticum durum)
Alcohol (Spirits—Specific Types)
Amp-Isostearoyl Hydrolyzed
    Wheat Protein
Atta Flour
Barley Grass (can contain seeds)
Barley Hordeum vulgare
Barley Malt
Beer (most contain barley or wheat)
Bleached Flour
Bran
Bread Flour
Brewer's Yeast
Brown Flour
Bulgur (Bulgar Wheat/Nuts)
Bulgur Wheat
Cereal Binding
Chilton
Club Wheat (Triticum aestivum
    subspecies compactum)
Common Wheat (Triticum aestivum)
Cookie Crumbs
Cookie Dough
Cookie Dough Pieces
Couscous
Crisped Rice
Dinkle (Spelt)
Disodium Wheatgermamido Peg-2
    Sulfosuccinate
Durum Wheat (Triticum durum)
Edible Coatings
Edible Films
Edible Starch
Einkorn (Triticum monococcum)
Emmer (Triticum dicoccon)
Enriched Bleached Flour
Enriched Bleached Wheat Flour
Enriched Flour
Farina
Farina Graham
Farro

Filler
Flour (normally this is wheat)
Fu (dried wheat gluten)
Germ
Graham Flour
Granary Flour
Groats (barley, wheat)
Hard Wheat
Heeng
Hing
Hordeum Vulgare Extract
Hydrolyzed Wheat Gluten
Hydrolyzed Wheat Protein
Hydrolyzed Wheat Protein Pg-Propyl
    Silanetriol
Hydrolyzed Wheat Starch
Hydroxypropyltrimonium Hydrolyzed
    Wheat Protein
Kamut (Pasta wheat)
Kecap Manis (Soy Sauce)
Ketjap Manis (Soy Sauce)
Kluski Pasta
Macha Wheat (Triticum aestivum)
Maida (Indian wheat flour)
Malt
Malt Extract
Malt Flavoring
Malt Syrup
Malt Vinegar
Malted Barley Flour
Malted Milk
Matza
Matzah
Matzo
Matzo Semolina
Meringue
Meripro 711
Mir
Nishasta
Oriental Wheat (Triticum turanicum)
Orzo Pasta
Pasta
Pearl Barley

Persian Wheat (Triticum carthlicum)
Perungayam
Polish Wheat (Triticum polonicum)
Poulard Wheat (Triticum turgidum)
Rice Malt (if barley or Koji are used)
Roux
Rusk
Rye
Seitan
Semolina
Semolina Triticum
Shot Wheat (Triticum aestivum)
Small Spelt
Spelt (Triticum spelta)
Spirits (Specific Types)
Sprouted Wheat or Barley
Stearyldimoniumhydroxypropyl
    Hydrolyzed Wheat Protein
Strong Flour
Suet in Packets
Tabbouleh
Tabouli
Teriyaki Sauce
Timopheevi Wheat (Triticum timopheevii)
Triticale X triticosecale
Triticum Vulgare (Wheat) Flour Lipids
Triticum Vulgare (Wheat) Germ Extract
Triticum Vulgare (Wheat) Germ Oil
Udon (wheat noodles)
Unbleached Flour
Vavilovi Wheat (Triticum aestivum)
Vital Wheat Gluten
Wheat, Abyssinian Hard (Triticum durum)
Wheat Amino Acids
Wheat Bran Extract
Wheat, Bulgur
Wheat Durum Triticum
Wheat Germ Extract
Wheat Germ Glycerides
Wheat Germ Oil
Wheat Germamidopropyldimonium
    Hydroxypropyl (Hydrolyzed Wheat
    Protein)

Wheat Grass (can contain seeds)
Wheat Nuts
Wheat Protein
Wheat (Triticum aestivum)
Wheat (Triticum monococcum)
Wheat (Triticum vulgare) Bran Extract
Whole-Meal Flour
Wild Einkorn (Triticum boeotictim)
Wild Emmer (Triticum dicoccoides)

The following items may or may not contain gluten depending on where and how they are made, and it is sometimes necessary to check with the manufacturer to find out:

Artificial Color[4]
Baking Powder[4]
Caramel Color[1,3]
Caramel Flavoring[1,3]
Clarifying Agents[4]
Coloring[4]
Dextrimaltose[1,7]
Dextrins[1,7]
Dry Roasted Nuts[4]
Emulsifiers[4]
Enzymes[4]
Fat Replacer[4]
Flavoring[6]
Food Starch[1,4]
Food Starch Modified[1,4]
Glucose Syrup[4]
Gravy Cubes[4]
Ground Spices[4]
HPP[4]
HVP[4]
Hydrogenated Starch Hydrolysate[4]
Hydrolyzed Plant Protein[4]
Hydrolyzed Protein[4]
Hydrolyzed Vegetable Protein[4]
Hydroxypropylated Starch[4]
Maltose[4]
Miso[4]
Mixed Tocopherols[4]

Modified Food Starch[1,4]
Modified Starch[1,4]
Natural Flavoring[6]
Natural Flavors[6]
Natural Juices[4]
Nondairy Creamer[4]
Pregelatinized Starch[4]
Protein Hydrolysates[4]
Seafood Analogs[4]
Seasonings[4]
Sirimi[4]
Smoke Flavoring[4]
Soba Noodles[4]
Soy Sauce[4]
Soy Sauce Solids[4]
Sphingolipids[4]
Stabilizers[4]
Starch[1,4]
Stock Cubes[4]
Suet[4]
Tocopherols[4]
Vegetable Broth[4]
Vegetable Gum[4]
Vegetable Protein[4]
Vegetable Starch[4]
Vitamins[4]
Wheat Starch[5]

1. If this ingredient is made in North America it is likely to be gluten free.
3. The problem with caramel color is it may or may not contain gluten depending on how it is manufactured. In the USA caramel color must conform with the FDA standard of identity from 21CFR CH.1. This statute says: the color additive caramel is the dark-brown liquid or solid material resulting from the carefully controlled heat treatment of the following food-grade carbohydrates: Dextrose (corn sugar), invert sugar, lactose (milk sugar), malt syrup (usually from barley malt), molasses (from cane), starch hydrolysates and fractions thereof (can include wheat), sucrose (cane or beet). Also, acids, alkalis, and salts are listed as additives which may be employed to assist the caramelization process.

4. Can utilize a gluten-containing grain or by-product in the manufacturing process, or as an ingredient.

5. Most celiac organizations in the USA and Canada do not believe that wheat starch is safe for celiacs. In Europe, however, <u>Codex Alimentarius Quality wheat starch</u> is considered acceptable in the celiac diet by most doctors and celiac organizations. This is a higher quality of wheat starch than is generally available in the USA or Canada.

6. According to 21 C.F.R. S 101,22(a)(3): "[t]he terms natural flavor or natural flavoring means the essential oil, oleoresin, essence or extractive, protein hydrolysate, distillate, or any product of roasting, heating or enzymolysis, which contains the flavoring constituents derived from a spice, fruit or fruit juice, vegetable or vegetable juice, edible yeast, herb, bark, bud, root, leaf or similar plant material, meat, seafood, poultry, eggs, dairy products, or fermentation products thereof. Whose significant function in food is flavoring rather than nutritional."

7. Dextrin is an incompletely hydrolyzed starch. It is prepared by dry heating corn, waxy maize, waxy milo, potato, arrowroot, WHEAT, rice, tapioca, or sago starches, or by dry heating the starches after: (1) Treatment with safe and suitable alkalis, acids, or pH control agents and (2) drying the acid or alkali treated starch. (1) Therefore, unless you know the source, you must avoid dextrin.

      May 1997 Sprue-Nik News.

      (1) Federal Register (4-1-96 Edition) 21CFR Ch.1, Section 184.12277. (2) Federal Register (4-1-96) 21 CFR. Ch.1, Section 184.1444

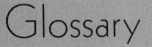

Glossary

Accommodation—A change made to the school, work, or other environment that will allow an individual with disabilities to succeed.

ADA—See Americans with Disabilities Act.

ADD—See Attention Deficit Disorder.

ADHD—See Attention Deficit Hyperactivity Disorder.

AGA—See Antigliadin Antibody.

Allergen—A substance that instigates an allergic reaction. See also Allergy; Histamine.

Allergy—A hypersensitivity or intolerance to a condition or substance (allergen) that spawns an adverse physiological reaction. See Histamine; Immunoglobulin E.

Americans with Disabilities Act (ADA)—The federal law that prohibits discrimination against people with disabilities in employment, public accommodations, and access to public facilities.

Amino Acid—One of the twenty-five organic acids that link together to form the proteins necessary for life.

Anemia—A condition in which the level of hemoglobin in the blood is too low. Often resulting from the malabsorption of iron, this condition is characterized by weakness, lethargy, and overall fatigue.

Anesthesiologist—A specialist who administers anesthesia, or medication that causes loss of sensation. Anesthesiologists are responsible for monitoring blood loss and vital signs, as well as pain management in sedated patients undergoing surgery. See also Conscious Sedation; Unconscious Sedation.

Antibody—A protein produced by the body that attaches to and kills antigens that threaten the body.

Antiendomysial Antibody (EmA)—One of the antibodies that a person with celiac disease produces when gluten is ingested. This antibody responds specifically to substances "attacking" the endomysium. It is one of the most important antibodies used for diagnosing celiac disease or detecting the presence of gluten in the diet.

Antigen—Invading organisms such as bacteria, viruses, fungi, or parasites that threaten the body. See also Antibody.

Antigliadin Antibody (AGA)—One of the antibodies that a person with celiac disease produces when gluten is ingested. Used for diagnosing celiac disease or detecting the presence of gluten in the diet.

Antihistamine—Medication used to counteract the effects of a histamine.

Antireticulin Antibody (ARA)—One of the antibodies that a person with celiac disease produces when gluten is ingested. Used for diagnosing celiac disease or detecting the presence of gluten in the diet.

ARA—See Antireticulin Antibody.

Asymptomatic—Showing few or no symptoms of a condition.

Asymptomatic Celiac Disease—Having celiac disease, but showing few or no symptoms of it. Many people with celiac disease are asymptomatic.

Atrophy—A wasting away; a diminution in the size of a cell, tissue, organ, or part.

Attention Deficit Disorder (ADD)—A condition characterized by inattention and distractibility, but not the hyperactivity seen in Attention Deficit Hyperactivity Disorder.

Attention Deficit Hyperactivity Disorder (ADHD)—A condition characterized by distractibility, restlessness, short attention span, impulsivity, and hyperactivity. See also Attention Deficit Disorder.

Autoimmune Disorder—The general term for a disorder in which the body's immune system produces antibodies against itself, the mistaken attack resulting in tissue damage. Celiac disease is an autoimmune disorder.

B-cell—A lymphocyte, or type of white blood cell, of the immune system responsible for making antibodies. Allergens are detected by B-cells in the blood. See also T-cell.

Biopsy—A procedure involving the removal of living tissue from the body to examine microscopically for the purpose of diagnosing disease.

"Bleed" Test—A procedure in which the finger is pricked with a needle and blood is squeezed out until the body naturally stops the flow.

B.R.A.T. Diet—Diet consisting of bananas, rice, apples, and dry toast, commonly recommended by pediatricians for children with diarrhea.

Calcium—An element taken in through the diet that is essential for a variety of bodily functions, such as neurotransmission, muscle contraction, and proper heart function. Commonly found in dairy products.

Casein— A protein found in milk and other dairy products. Casein may also be present in many prepared foods, including hot dogs, sausages, baked goods, nutrition bars, salad dressing, sherbet, and milk chocolate. Note that a food that is lactose free is not necessarily casein free.

CD—See Celiac Disease.

Celiac Disease (CD)—A genetic autoimmune disorder in which gluten intolerance leads to damage to the lining of the small intestine. The incidence is estimated at approximately 1 in 150 to 1 in 250 people worldwide. Also known as coeliac disease, gluten-sensitive enteropathy, and nontropical sprue.

Cell—The smallest unit of a living organism; the basic structure for tissues and organs.

Central Nervous System—Made up of the brain and spinal cord, this system is responsible for controlling what we think and do.

Chronic Diarrhea—Ongoing, recurrent diarrhea.

Chronic Fatigue Syndrome—A condition of prolonged and severe tiredness or weariness (fatigue) that is not relieved by rest and is not directly caused by other conditions.

Coeliac Disease—Alternate spelling of celiac disease.

Compensated-Latent Disease—A form of celiac disease in which the condition is present, but not visible or active.

Conscious Sedation—Light sedation during which the patient retains airway reflexes and can respond when spoken to. See also Anesthesiologist; Unconscious Sedation.

Constipation—Condition in which stools are excessively firm and difficult to excrete during infrequent bowel movements.

Crohn's Disease—An inflammatory bowel disease characterized by scarring of the small intestine and/or colon due to chronic inflammation of the digestive tract. Characterized by diarrhea, abdominal pain, and sometimes blood in the stool.

Dermatitis Herpetiformis (DH)—A disorder, closely related to celiac disease, caused by intolerance to gluten and characterized by external manifestations (rash) as well as damage to the small intestine.

DH—See Dermatitis Herpetiformis.

Diabetes—An autoimmune disease characterized by excessive urination and excessive thirst. There are two types: diabetes insipidus is caused by a pituitary deficiency; diabetes mellitus involves an insulin deficiency.

Diarrhea—Loose stools during excessively frequent bowel movements. See also Chronic Diarrhea.

Disability—A term used to describe a delay in physical, cognitive, social, and/or emotional development.

Discrimination—Showing favor toward one person, race, or group and prejudice toward another.

Distended—Swollen due to pressure within. A distended abdomen is a common symptom of celiac disease.

Dominant Trait—A characteristic or condition a child inherits because a dominant gene for that trait overrides any recessive gene it has been paired with. See also Recessive Trait.

EmA—See Antiendomysial Antibody.

Endomysial—Involving the endomysium.

Endomysium—A sheath of connective tissue that surrounds muscle fibers. In people with celiac disease, the antiendomysial antibody responds specifically to substances "attacking" the endomysium in the intestine.

Endoscope—A narrow, flexible tube inserted into the body when performing an endoscopy. The endoscope is lighted and usually has a small clipper that can remove tissue samples.

Endoscopy—A procedure in which an endoscope is inserted into a body cavity for visual examination. For the purpose of diagnosing celiac disease, the endoscope is threaded through the mouth to the small intestine, where a doctor removes tissue samples that are later sent to a lab for biopsy.

Enzyme—A protein that speeds up a chemical change in the body, such as in the digestion of foods.

Epilepsy—A condition characterized by recurrent seizures (muscle contractions or changes in consciousness) that are caused by abnormal electrical activity in the brain.

Failure to Thrive—Describes a condition in which a child experiences below-average weight-gain or below-average increase in height.

False Negative—A test result that incorrectly indicates no disease.

Fatty Stool Test—Used to confirm the presence of celiac disease, a stool is examined for high fat content indicated by buoyancy. See also Steatorrhea.

Folic Acid—The synthetic form of folate, a B vitamin found naturally in many foods and important for the formation of red and white blood cells.

"Free Appropriate Public Education"—The right, under IDEA, of every child with disabilities to an education provided at public expense that is appropriate to his or her developmental strengths and needs.

Gastroenterologist—A physician specializing in medical problems associated with the digestive system; qualified to diagnose and supervise the treatment of celiac disease.

Gastrointestinal—Relating to the stomach and intestines.

Gastrointestinal Distress—The experience of cramping, bloating, gas, or diarrhea.

Gene—The basic unit of heredity that transmits particular traits such as eye color from parent to child, located at specific points on chromosomes, made up of DNA and protein.

Genetic—Inherited.

"Genetic Fingerprint"—See Human Leukocyte Antigen.

Genotype—The inherited characteristics of an individual, as determined by the complete set of genes on his or her chromosomes.

GF—See Gluten-Free.

Gliadin—The part of the protein in gluten-containing grains that is soluble in alcohol; the promaline portion of the gluten molecule. The type of reaction an individual with celiac disease experiences may be determined by the amount of gliadin in a given food.

Glutelin—A simple protein found in the seeds of cereal grains; a component of gluten. See also Promaline.

Gluten—A protein found in wheat, rye, barley, and oats.

Gluten Antibody Blood Test—See Serum Antibody Test.

Gluten-Free (GF)—Containing no gluten.

Gluten Intolerance—An inability to properly digest foods containing gluten.

Gluten-Sensitive Enteropathy (GSE)—Another name for celiac disease.

GSE—See Gluten-Sensitive Enteropathy.

Gut—An intestine; a bowel; the whole alimentary canal (from mouth to anus).

Hemorrhage—Heavy bleeding from a blood vessel.

Histamine—The chemical compound that causes the disagreeable symptoms of an allergic reaction. See also Allergen; Allergy; Antihistamine.

HLA—See Human Leukocyte Antigen.

Human Leukocyte Antigen (HLA)—A protein that protrudes from the surface of a person's cells. The HLAs, which make up the "genetic fingerprint," allow the immune cells in the body to recognize things that belong specifically to that person.

IBS—See Irritable Bowel Syndrome.

IDEA—See Individuals with Disablilities Education Act.

IEP—See Individualized Education Program.

IgA—See Immunoglobulin A.

IgE—See Immunoglobulin E.

IgG—See Immunoglobulin G.

Immune System—The complicated network of molecules that produce antibodies, which eliminate infections caused by bacteria, viruses, and invading microbes, defending the body against disease.

Immunoglobulin A (IgA)—Present in the secretions of the body's mucous membranes, this is one of the antibodies that a person with celiac disease produces when gluten is ingested. Used for diagnosing celiac disease or detecting the presence of gluten in the diet. See also Antigliadin Antibody.

Immunoglobulin E (IgE)—One of the antibodies produced in response to an allergen that a person with celiac disease makes when gluten is ingested. Used for diagnosing celiac disease or detecting the presence of gluten in the diet.

Immunoglobulin G (IgG)—The primary type of antibody that responds to invading organisms in the body. It is one of the antibodies that a person with celiac disease produces when gluten is ingested. Used for diagnosing celiac disease or detecting the presence of gluten in the diet. See also Antigliadin Antibody.

Individualized Education Program (IEP)—In the U.S., the written plan that specifies the special education goals and the services the local education agency has agreed to provide a child with disabilities who is eligible under IDEA; for children ages three to twenty-one.

Individuals with Disabilities Education Act (IDEA)—A federal law originally passed in 1975 and subsequently amended that requires states to provide a "free appropriate public education in the least restrictive environment" to children with disabilities.

Infertility—The inability to conceive offspring.

Inherited—Relating to traits, such as eye and hair color or certain conditions, passed through genes from one generation to another. Used synonymously with genetic.

Intestine—The passageway from the stomach to the anus, consisting of the large and small intestines, through which food travels and is digested.

Irritable Bowel Syndrome (IBS)—A functional bowel disorder characterized by recurrent cramping, abdominal pain, and diarrhea.

Lactase—An enzyme produced in the small intestine that breaks lactose into two simpler sugars, thereby helping the body to digest lactose.

Lactose—A sugar found in dairy products that can cause an allergic reaction. See also Allergy; Lactase; Lactose Intolerance.

Lactose Intolerance—An inability to tolerate lactose, which can result in gastrointestinal distress. Sometimes caused by an interruption in the production of lactase. Common in people with untreated celiac disease.

Latent—Present but inactive.

Leaky Gut Syndrome—A condition in which damage to, or differences in, the intestinal lining may allow partially digested food or other matter from the intestine to leak out into the bloodstream. Also known as intestinal permeability.

Lupus—An autoimmune disorder in which the body develops antibodies against the DNA of its own cells, resulting in abnormalities of blood vessels and connective tissue.

Lymphocytes—White blood cells of the immune system, lymphocytes are divided into two major classes: B-cells and T-cells.

Lymphoma—Encompassing a variety of cancers of the lymphatic system, lymphoma is characterized by the uncontrollable multiplication of lymph cells resulting in symptoms such as swelling of the lymph nodes, itching, fatigue, weight-loss, and fever. People with celiac disease are 40 to 100 times more likely to develop intestinal lymphoma than those unaffected.

Malabsorption—Inefficient absorption of nutrients from food as it passes from the mouth through the esophagus, stomach, and intestines to the anus. Results in malnourishment.

Malnourishment—The state of being improperly nourished or sustained by the substances necessary for life and growth.

Molecule—The smallest particle of an element or compound that can exist in the free state and still maintain its recognizable characteristics.

Mucosal Damage—Injury to the mucous membrane, or lining, of body cavities.

Multigenetic—Describes a condition in which several genes, perhaps each having different strengths of expression, are involved in contributing to a specific trait. Celiac disease is believed to be multigenetic. See also Dominant Trait; Recessive Trait.

Negative Predictive Value—The probability of no disease in a patient with a negative test result. See also Positive Predictive Value.

Nontropical Sprue—Another name for celiac disease.

Osteomalacia—A condition caused by vitamin D deficiency, leading to the loss of calcium from bones. This, in turn, can result in weakened bones or fractures. The same condition in children is called rickets.

Osteoporosis—A reduction in the amount of bone mass, so that fractures can occur after minimal trauma.

Pediatric Gastroenterologist (Pediatric G.I.)—A gastroenterologist whose patients are children.

Pediatric G.I.—See Pediatric Gastroenterologist.

Phytonutrients—Certain chemical components found naturally in plants that are believed to enhance human health. Examples of phytonutrients include: carotenoids (found in carrots, tomatoes, citrus and some other fruits, and green leafy vegetables) and flavonoids (found in many fruits and wines).

Phlebotomist—A professional who draws blood using a needle and tourniquet.

Positive Predictive Value—The probability of disease in a patient with a positive test result. See also Negative Predictive Value.

Prolamine—A simple protein found in plants that cannot be dissolved in anything except strong alcohol solutions. It is an important component of gluten. Also spelled prolamin. See also Gliadin; Glutelin.

Protein—An organic compound, made up of linked amino acids, necessary for life.

Recessive Trait—A characteristic or condition that is inherited only when the gene for that trait is transmitted to the offspring by both parents. See also Dominant Trait.

Rehabilitation Act of 1973—Section 504 of this federal law prohibits discrimination against individuals with disabilities in federally funded programs.

Reticulin—Constituent protein of reticular fibers: collagen type III.

Rickets—A childhood disease caused by a vitamin D deficiency. Characterized by abnormalities in the shape and structure of bones, body tenderness, sweating of the head, and an enlarged liver and spleen. See also Osteomalacia.

Section 504—See Rehabilitation Act of 1973.

Sensitivity—The probability of a positive test result in a patient with disease. See also Specificity.

Serological Test—A blood test.

Serum Antibody Test—A blood test that detects the presence of antibodies to a particular antigen. In celiac disease, the test can provide evidence of gluten in the body. Also known as Gluten Antibody Blood Test.

Small Intestine—Extending from the stomach to the large intestine, the small intestine is composed of three sections: duodenum, jejunum, and ileum. All are involved in the absorption of nutrients. In celiac disease, the duodenum is first to be affected.

Specificity—The probability of a negative test result in a patient without disease. See also Sensitivity.

Steatorrhea—A condition, characterized by foul, frothy, sometimes floating stools, in which there is an abnormally large amount of fat in the stool; usually the result of poor absorption in the small intestine as in celiac disease. See also Fatty Stool Test.

Symptom—An indication of a disease or disorder that is noticed by a patient and can help in reaching a diagnosis.

T-cell—A critical lymphocyte, or type of white blood cell, of the immune system that aids in destroying infected cells and coordinates the overall immune response.

Thyroid Disease—A disease of the thyroid gland, which secretes hormones important for controlling body metabolism. "Hypothyroid" describes an underactive thyroid gland; "hyperthyroid" describes an overactive thyroid gland.

Tissue Transglutaminase (tTG)—A blood test that measures EmA-IgA levels. Very specific to detecting the presence of antibodies released by people with celiac disease when gluten is ingested.

tTG—See Tissue Transglutaminase.

Unconscious Sedation—Sedation in which the patient is completely "asleep" during surgery. See also Anesthesiologist; Conscious Sedation.

Villi—Small hair-like projections on certain mucous membranes in the body that secrete mucus and absorb nutrients from digested food. People with celiac disease can become malnourished and dehydrated if the villi in the intestine are damaged by gluten and cannot perform their function.

Vitamin D—The "sunshine vitamin" produced by the body when exposed to UV light. Plays an important role in calcium and phosphorus metabolism. See also Osteomalacia; Rickets.

White Blood Cell—One of three types of blood cells. They protect the body by destroying harmful or foreign substances such as bacteria, viruses, and fungi.

Zonulin—Recently discovered in high levels in individuals with celiac disease, this protein opens the spaces between cells, allowing some substances to pass through, while preventing harmful bacteria and toxins from entering.

Index